ADVANCES IN LAPAROSCOPIC SURGERY

Edited by **Arshad M. Malik**

Advances in Laparoscopic Surgery
Edited by Arshad M. Malik

Published by InTech
Janeza Trdine 9, 51000 Rijeka, Croatia

Publishing Process Manager Maja Kisic

Technical Editor Teodora Smiljanic

Cover Designer InTech Design Team

Additional hard copies can be obtained from orders@intechopen.com

Advances in Laparoscopic Surgery, Edited by Arshad M. Malik
p. cm.
ISBN 978-953-307-933-2

For EU product safety concerns:
IN TECH d.o.o., Prolaz Marije Krucifikse Kozulić 3, 51000 Rijeka, Croatia,
info@intechopen.com or visit our website at intechopen.com.

Meet the editor

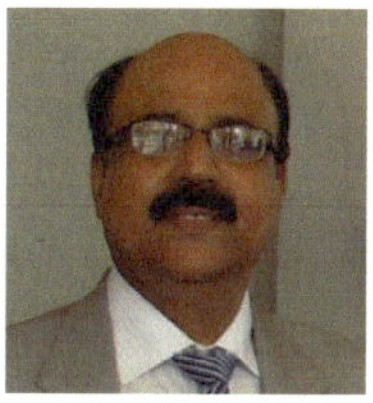

Dr Arshad M. Malik is presently working as Associate Professor of Surgery at the College of Medicine, Qassim University, Kingdom of Saudi Arabia. He is the author of about 30 scientific papers, of which 21 are published in international journals. He has presented 18 podium presentations at international conferences, including USA, Berlin, Spain, Hong Kong, Seoul, Bali, Vietnam, Singapore, and in many other places like India and China. His presentations are much appreciated and well received by the leaders in this field. He has attended about 30 international conferences nationally and abroad as well. Dr Malik is very keen to further his knowledge and skills by way of attending workshops at the international and national level on laparo-endoscopic surgery. He is also the supervisor of FCPS trainees, and presently training three candidates in this field. He is very instrumental in organizing clinical meetings in his department, where he has been serving for many years.

Contents

Preface

There has been a tremendous change in the outlook of surgical patients ever since laparoscopic surgery has come into practice. Surgeons all over the world have seen this change, for which there is a great deal of enthusiasm, and have shown an eagerness to learn this novel technique. Laparoscopic surgery has passed through different stages of evolution to reach its present status where it has earned the title of "Gold Standard" treatment for various surgical problems. The initial period of the learning curve has now been shortened substantially, and most centers are imparting training to budding surgeons all over the world. It has also become an integral part of the curriculum of surgical training in most degree/diploma-awarding institutes globally.

There were days when the scope of laparoscopic surgery was very limited, but improved skills, experience, and advancement in instrumentation has brought a phenomenal change so that there are hardly any contraindications to laparoscopic surgery left. Laparoscopic surgery is praised by surgeons and patients alike in terms of the length of hospital stay, pain, and overall cost. There is also an improvement in the cosmetic results of surgery evidenced by a scar of 10 centimeters, compared to virtually no scar at all. We have seen a parallel rise in the efficiency of surgeons as more and more surgeons have stepped into this new world of advanced technology.

This book is intended to highlight the advancements in the technique and scope of laparoscopic surgery. A number of new therapeutic, as well as diagnostic procedures, are being shared by many experts in this field. I hope that this book will be a lot of help for trainees, as well as those practicing laparoscopic surgery, to improve their knowledge and skills by sharing the experience of the people who have contributed to this book. My special thanks go to all the authors who were able to spare their valuable and precious time. I look forward to any suggestions for improvement on this book, and welcome any positive criticism to help improve upon this book in future.

December 01, 2011

Dr Arshad M. Malik
Liaquat University Of Medical and Health Sciences, Sindh,
Pakistan

Part 1

General Surgery Procedures

1

The Laparoscopic Appendectomy – A Recent Trend

Arshad M. Malik
Liaquat University of Medical and Health Sciences, Jamshoro (Sindh), Pakistan

1. Introduction

Acute appendicitis is one of the commonest surgical problems afflicting a major population all over the world. No age is immune to it but it is most prevalent during adolescent and child hood. The outcome can be very serious at both extremes of life and there is a life time risk of developing acute appendicitis in about 5-8% nothing. An early surgical removal after diagnosis is the most preferred and agreeable treatment. Appendectomy through grid iron incision has enjoyed a unique reputation of a standard operation globally. It is one of the most common abdominal operations performed all over the world. The open appendectomy through right grid iron incision was introduced by Mc Burney (Mc Burney 1894) and this technique enjoyed decades of un-opposed reputation and widespread use globally because of its proven safety and efficacy. The introduction of laparoscopy has brought a major change in the field of surgery. The laparoscopic appendectomy is gradually gaining popularity over the past 10-15 years by way of proving improved diagnostic outcome and decreased rate of wound problems. It was way back in 1983 when a first laparoscopic surgery for acute appendicitis was performed by a German Gynaecologist Semm (Semm K 1983). There are a number of reports published in favour of laparoscopic approach in terms of rapid recovery, a faster wound healing, lowered rate of complications, and an early resumption of oral intake (Martin LC et al 1995) while others (John Brenden Hansen 1996) claimed that though it takes a comparatively longer time but yet is safe and effective way of treating acute appendicitis as it reduces post-operative stay substantially and would help the patient return to work earlier. An almost similar recommendation came from many similar studies in a very short span of time comparing laparoscopic versus open appendectomy, claiming substantial advantage over open technique (Rober Globus et al 1998). A superiority in terms of cosmetic results and cost-effectiveness was another reason that majority favoured this recently introduced technique. A recent study claims it to be a safe option in children compared to the open operation (Lee SL 2011). There were however a lot of reservations as to the safety and applicability of this procedure as elaborated by many studies (Ingraham et al 2010) (Yano H et al 2004) (Kamal M 2003). There is a limitation to the use of this laparoscopic approach in third world countries where the economical constraints, lack of facility and a general fear keeps them from getting operated (Saunders S 2002). Despite all the limitations ,the scope of laparoscopic appendectomy is on the rise and although it has not yet achieved the status of a "Gold Standard " treatment as enjoyed by laparoscopic cholecystectomy, there is a gradual acceptance of this procedure all over the world based on various factors in favour of laparoscopic approach. The main advantages reported over open appendectomy include an accuracy of diagnosis especially in females when various other conditions can mimic acute appendicitis, an excellent cosmetic outcome, minimal tissue trauma, substantially reduced operative and post operative complications, and an early return to work. Ulrich Guller et al 2004 proposed that laparoscopic appendectomy decreases in-hospital admission, in hospital mortality, and post operative complications. Despite innumerable reports favouring laparoscopic appendectomy, the technique is really slow to gain popularity and not many centres are doing this procedure regularly. There seems to be no obvious reasons for this. The uptake of laparoscopic technique for appendicitis is slow to evolve all over the world. Loannis Kehagias et al 2008 reported recently very promising results of laparoscopic appendectomy emphasizing availability of the sophisticated instruments as well as adequate experience of the surgeon to play a key role for a successful laparoscopic appendectomy. The elderly patients are thought to be at a higher risk of developing complications following acute appendicitis and there are reports claiming that laparoscopic appendectomy is a presumably superior option for the elderly victims of acute appendicitis (Wu SC et al 2011). Despite of lots of benefits elaborated in many randomized trials and other similar studies talking high of laparoscopic approach, a number of critics have shown a marginal benefit of the laparoscopic approach over open conventional technique (Jane Garbutt 1999, Kathouda N 2005, Oannis Kehagias 2008, Olmi S 2995, Lee SL 2011, Saunders S 2002, Martin LC, 1995,). The adequate data in favour of this technique has not really brought a significant change of mind as yet and there is a clear split of opinion as to the optimum method of treatment of acute appendicitis. There is a school of thought which considers this mode of treatment to be time consuming, but shorter hospital stay, better cosmetic results and cost effective. This is contrary to the belief of many surgeons who continue to practice open appendectomy by the same conventional method considering it to be the standard operation for acute appendicitis. The real challenge in laparoscopic approach is considered to be those patients where the appendix is severely inflamed, twisted, retro-caecal or is in pelvis or there are firm adhesions making its skeletinization difficult by laparoscopic means. It is claimed that the commonest problems faced are in the complicated appendicitis where even the experts feel difficulty. A number of conflicting results negating the advocates were published making its feasibility questionable in complicated cases of acute appendicitis (Ortega AE et al 1995) (Bresciani et al 2005) (Katkhuda N 2005). Yoshiwa et all claim lack of proper training and lack of knowledge about basic technique to be responsible for its limited use presently . An extended and undue prolonged operative time taken in laparoscopic approach has been reported to be one of the disadvantages of this technique (Reiertsen O etal 1997). This has been attributed to the learning curve of the surgeons and it was believed that with experience the difference in operative time of the two techniques becomes almost negligible (Kehagias I et al 2008). Similarly, the cost effectiveness can be achieved by decreasing the operative time and a high level of skill to make it more feasible for the developing countries (Ali R et al 2010).The laparoscopic procedure is still under evaluation and a number of changes are made in the original procedure. Vipul D et al introduced a two port technique instead of three port technique introduced, (Song Yi Kim et al 2010). This report was carried out by a trainee and there was a learning curve of thirty patients. (Ulritch Guller et al 2004) proposed laparoscopic appendectomy to be much superior than the open technique in terms of hospital stay, cosmetics, early return to work and post-operative mortality. There are reports questioning its cost as there is longer operative time and use of disposable instruments, multiplying the actual cost manyfolds compared to the open appendectomy (Ignacio RC 2004). This is contrary to the belief of others (Neendham PJ et al 2009) who claim that laparoscopic appendectomy can be performed in a reasonable cost despite use of disposable items. Despite accumulation of substantial data favouring laparoscopic appendectomy, there continues an expanding controversy as to the safety if this procedure in patients with complicated appendicitis as well as post-operative recovery and operative time.

2. Guidelines for laparoscopic appendectomy

There are certain guidelines as laid down by the experts who are considered pioneers of various laparoscopic procedures. These guidelines would help the beginners to follow so as to avoid any undue stress and mistakes during the early phase of their training. These guidelines are based on the existing data coupled with individual experiences formed into consensus. These guidelines help the beginners to have a better understanding of the procedure as to the proper selection of the patients, the indications of laparoscopic appendectomy, various complications that might develop and thus to select the most appropriate operative procedure under a given situation. The best guidelines in this regard are provided by the society of American Gastro-intestinal and Endoscopic Surgeons (SAGES). A similar guideline focussing on diagnosis and treatment of acute appendicitis is provided by SSAT (Society for the surgery of alimentary tract).

3. Verities of laparoscopic appendectomy

The laparoscopic appendectomy is divided into two basic approaches as under

1. Intra-corporeal Laparoscopic appendectomy
2. Extra-Corporeal appendectomy.

The intra-corporeal variety involves the creation of pneumo-peritoneum by a 10mm supra-umbilical port followed by the insertion two 5mm working ports well outside the midline. A thorough inspection of the abdominal cavity is followed by identification, skeletinization and removal of the appendix after ligation/clipping of the meso-appendix intra-corporeally. This approach is adopted and practiced at a number of centres and is gradually gaining reputation as a good alternative to the open appendectomy.

The extra-corporeal video assisted appendectomy is another type of laparoscopic appendectomy which involves the initial steps of intracorporeal appendectomy up till creation of pneumo-peritoneum, identification and skeletinization of appendix same as in the case of intra-corporeal appendectomy. The following steps differ in that the appendix is brought out on the surface through a 10 mm port in right iliac fossa and then further steps are just the same as in open appendectomy. This technique usually involves 2-3 ports (Konstadoulakis MM et al 2004) but a number of studies have recently published using the same technique with a single peri-umbilical port (Koontz CS et al 2006). The author compared video-assisted extra-corporeal appendectomy with conventional open appendectomy believing that this method has an advantage over open appendectomy of having less chances of diagnostic error as well as it has the advantages of open appendectomy of feeling the appendix, ligating the appendix manually outside on the surface . This has an additional advantage of having a secure ligation of meso- appendix to avoid cystic arterial bleeding. Before displaying the results of the study, a brief introduction to the basic technique of video-assisted extra-corporeal appendectomy (VAECA) is given below.

3.1 Technique of video-assisted laparoscopic appendectomy (Malik et al 2009)

This is a modified form of laparoscopic appendectomy where we combine the steps of both open and inta-corporeal techniques of appendectomy. The surgeon stands on left side of the supine patient. A 10 mm sub-umbilical port is made for the camera while another 10 mm port is made in the right iliac fossa. Both of these ports can be interchanged for camera as and when needed. The identification and skeletinization of the appendix is much easier because of video-scopic vision where surgeon can actually visualize if there are any adhesions and a finger guided adhesiolysis can be done under vision. Once the appendix is identified and isolated, a grasper is introduced to get hold of the organ and the abdominal cavity is deflated and appendix is drawn on the surface. The remaining steps are just as the way we perform open appendectomy. Once the meso-appendix is ligated and appendix removed, the appendicular stump is returned back and ports are closed after a final look inside the abdominal cavity.Some of the steps of this procedure are highlighted below by the following operative pictures

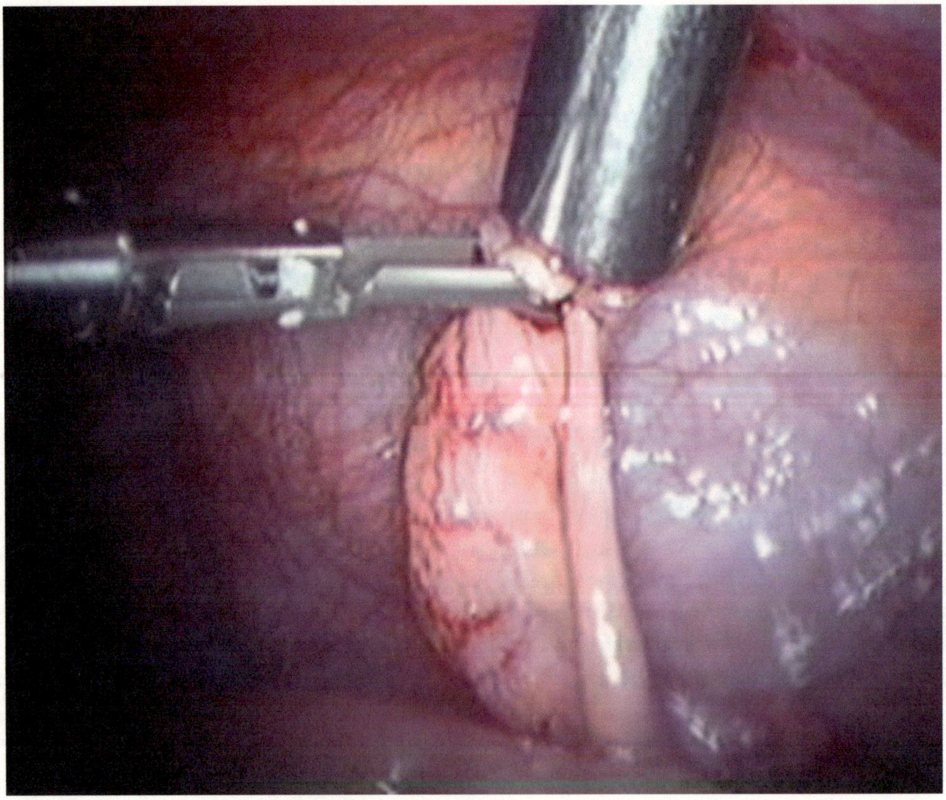

Fig. 1. Appendix drawn into sheath of 10mm trocar

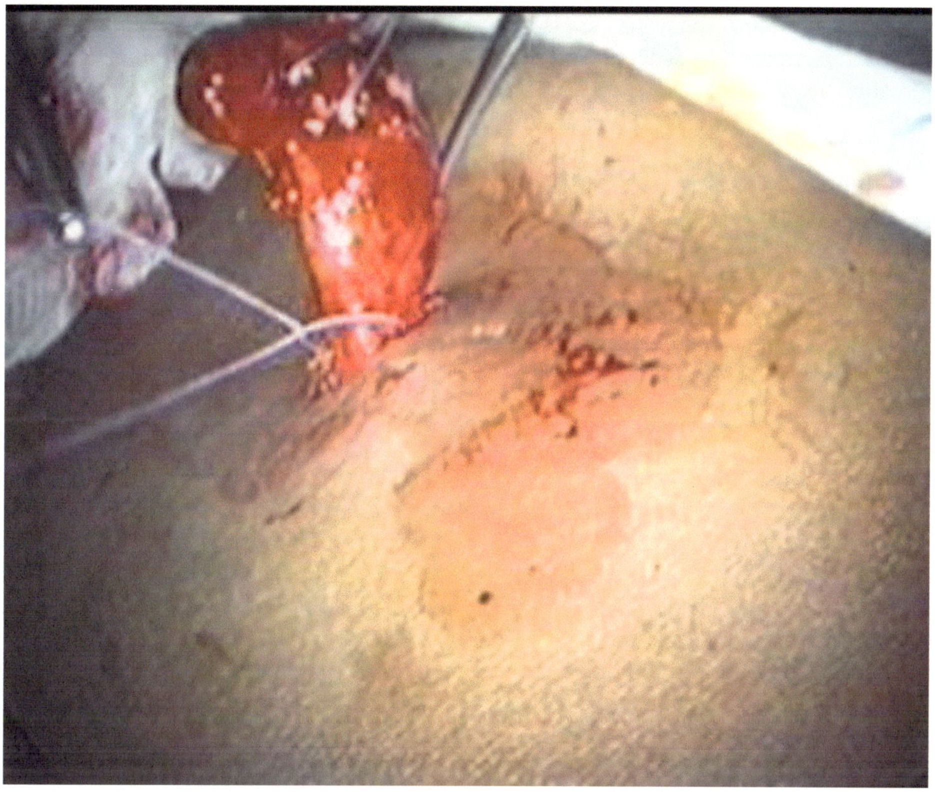

Fig. 2. Appendix drawn out on surface and meson-appendix legated.

3.2 Authors study

Author conducted a study in 2009 comparing the open appendectomy (OA) versus Video assisted extra-corporeal appendectomy (VAECA) wherein a total number of 283 patients of acute appendicitis were split into two groups. We explained this newly emerging technique as well as the conventional appendectomy to all the patients as and when they were diagnosed. The intended operative techniques were fully explained to the patients in terms of merits and demerits of the operative technique. The grouping of the patients was based on their own choice and by coin toss when patients did not show any preference for any particular technique. Of the total number, 150(53%) were operated by open Technique while 133(47%) by video-assisted extracorporeal technique of appendectomy. Majority of patients (89%) in the VAECA group were operated by three port technique while few (11%) could be successfully completed by two ports only. All patients below 10 years and those with suspected appendicular mass were excluded from the study. This was an initial study on the video assisted technique and we had promising results to conclude that VAECA could be a better alternate to open appendectomy in a majority of patients with acute appendicitis without complications. Some of the results are shown below showing comparison of the two techniques.

The results in our study were very promising in terms of safety, reliability and feasibility. The major advantages that we could conclude was fewer wound infections, less severe postoperative pain, better cosmesis, shorter operative time and early recovery. It was also compared in terms of cost as we found out that there is reasonable reduction in the total cost of operation in VAECA group because we ligated the mesoappendix and appendicular stump by a suture in place of metal clips usually applied in intracorporeal technique of laparoscopic appendectomy. The magnificent telescopic vision of whole abdomen makes identification and dissection of inflamed appendix reasonably easier compared to open appendectomy. It is claimed that VAECA combines safety and efficiency of both intracorporeal laparoscopic appendectomy and conventional open appendectomy (Valioulis I et al 2001). Any associated pathology can also be identified by using video assisted technique and this is of particular significance when diagnosis of acute appendicitis is doubtful (Mayer A et al 2004). The lowered rate of wound sepsis in our study are because of least contact of infected appendix with the surrounding walls of the port as it is fully drawn into the sheath of the trocar before its retrieval. This is contrary to the belief of Suttie SA and Seth S who claim an increased rate of wound infection in video-assisted extra-corporeal appendectomy compared to conventional open appendectomy (Suttie SA and Seth S 2004). Author continued the same study and a total number of the study subjects has reached to 1700 of which only 625(36.76%) gave consent for open appendectomy while remaining (63.23%, n=1075) patients were willing for video-assisted laparoscopic appendectomy. This clearly shows that the results of video-assisted laparoscopic appendectomy are more acceptable to the patients. There was a gross difference in the total operative time compared to the open conventional appendectomy as well as intra-corporeal appendectomy. The diagnostic error as well as confirmation of the diagnosis is more reliable in the video-assisted extra-corporeal appendectomy. The total cost is reduced in VAECA due to use of suture in place of clips and reduced operative time also adds reducing the cost of operation. Post-operative complications are reasonably less in VAECA compared to other two techniques of appendectomy. Author is convinced that video-assisted approach of laparoscopic appendectomy is a better alternative procedure that can be effective when there is simple acute appendicitis without mass formation or many adhesions. Further RCT's on this technique of VAECA can help establishing this technique as a better alternate in un-complicated patients of acute appendicitis and more so in young adult females where the diagnosis of acute appendicitis cannot be established with certainty.

	Type of operation (n = 283)		P value
	OA n (%)	VAECA n (%)	
Operative time:			
• Up to 30 minutes	14(9.3%)	95(71.4%)	
• 31-60 minutes	99(66.0%)	33(24.8%)	
• 61-90 minutes	31(20.7%)	3(2.3%)	
• Over 90 minutes	6(4.0%)	2(1.5%)	

*P value is <0.001 for all groups and is statistically highly significant
N= Number of the patients

Table 1. Comparison of mean operative time in both groups.

	Type of operation (n = 283)		P-Value
	OA n (%)	VAECA n (%)	
Operative problems:			
• Bleeding from appendicular artery	3(2.0%)	7(5.3%)	*< 0.001
• Perforation of appendix during mobilization	6(4.0%)	9(6.8%)	
• Lengthening of incision	32(21.3%)	4(3.0%)	
• Minor trauma to neighboring structures	2(1.3%)	5(3.8%)	
• Difficulty in mobilization	17(11.3%)	23(17.3%)	
• Difficulty in localization of appendix	19(12.7%)	7(5.3%)	

* *P value* is statistically highly significant for all groups
N= Number of patients

Table 2. Comparison of operative complications in both groups

	Type of operation (n = 283)		P value
	OA n (%)	VAECA n (%)	
Minor wound / port infection	13(8.7%)	7(5.3%)	< 0.01*
Partial wound dehiscence	9(6.0%)	0	
Wound/port bleeding	3(2.0%)	5(3.8%)	
Respiratory tract infection	13(8.7%)	7(5.3%)	
Residual abscess	5(3.3%)	2(1.5%)	

* *P value* is statistically significant
N= Number of patients

Table 3. Postoperative complications

	Type of operation (n = 283)		P value
	OA n (%)	VAECA n (%)	
1-2 days	66(44.0%)	128(96.2%)	< 0.001*
3-4 days	42(28.0%)	1(0.8%)	
5-6 days	42(28.0%)	4 (3.0%)	

* *P value* is statistically highly significant
N= Number of patients

Table 4. Hospital stays in both groups

4. Recent advances in laparoscopic appendectomy

During the last few years there has been a dramatic improvement in the techniques of gaining access to the abdominal cavity minimizing the number of ports to a single incision in order to improve the cosmetic results. A number of techniques such as single incision laparoscopic surgery (SILS) and natural orifice transluminal surgery(NOTES) are introduced to improve the outcome of minimal access surgery and to make it still further less traumatic to the patients. The same advancements also apply to the laparoscopic appendectomy to make it more and less traumatic by way of reducing the number of ports. Initially both intr-corporeal and extra-corporeal techniques were performed by two to three ports. Recently a single incision, multi-luminal port appendectomy is introduced. The safety and efficacy of these newer techniques is yet to be established as there are no Randomized control studies to claim their benefits over multi port laparoscopic appendectomy (Rehman H 2011). Roberts KE(2009) described a true single port appendectomy (TSPA) by a new technique which he describes as "puppeteer technique" using single port and a pully of thread pulling the appendix. He claims this technique to be first of its kind which reduces the minimal access surgery to a further minimum level. Ates et al 2007 described a similar single port technique successfully and claim that this single port technique further makes minimally invasive surgery a better and safe option with minimal tissue trauma. Natural orifice transluminal endoscopic surgery (NOTES) is the most recent advancement in laparoscopic surgery. A cadaveric model appendectomy using NOTES technique by Santos BF et al 2011 via anterior transrectal route is found to be feasible ,time saving and easier to perform compared to posterior rectal approach. Eung Jin Shin et al 2010 reported transvaginal appendectomy using NOTES indicating many limitations to its use in human beings.Although there has been a tremendous improvement and advancement in minimally invasive surgical techniques to improve the outcome of different surgical procedures in terms of cosmetic results and cost effectiveness but the final word about there efficacy and effectiveness is yet to be established.

5. References

Ali R, Khan MR, Pishori T, Tayyab M. Laparoscopic appendectomy for acute appendicitis. Is this a feasible option for developing countries? Saudi J Gastroenterol 2010; 16(1):25-29.

Ates O, Hakguder G, Olguner M, Akgur FM. Single-port laparoscopic appendectomy conducted intra-corporeally with the aid of a transabdominal sling suture. J Pediatr Surg 2007;42(6):1071-4.

Bresciani C, Perez RO, Habr-gama A, Jacob CE, Ozaki A, Batagello C et al. Laparoscopic versus standard appendectomy outcomes and cost comparison in the private sector. J gastrointestinal Surg 2005; 9:1174-80.

Chung RS, Rowland DY, Li P, Diaz J. A metaanalysis of randomized controlled trials of laparoscopic versus convention appendectomy. Am J Surg 1999; 177:250-53

Emple LK, Litwin DE, McLeods RS. A Meta analysis pf laparoscopic versus open appendectomy inpatients suspected of having acute appendicitis. Ca J Surg 1999; 42: 377-83.

Heinzelmann M, Simmen HP, Cummins, Laeriader F. Is laparoscopic appendectomy the new Gold standard? Arch surg 1995; 130(70); 782-85.

Hansen JB, , Smithers BM, Schache D, Wall DRMiller BM, Schache, Wall Dr. Laparoscopic versus open appendectomy. A randomized trial. World J Surg 1996; 20(1):17-21.

Ignacio Rc,Burke R, Spencer D,Bissel C, Dorsainvi C,Lucha PA.Laparoscopic versus open appendectomy.What is the real difference? Results of a prospective randomized double blinded trial. Surg Endos 2004; 18:334-337.

Ingraham AM, Cohen ME, Bjlimoria KY, Pritts Ta, Ko CY, Esposito TJ. Comparison of outcomes after laparoscopic versus open appendectomy for acute appendicitis at 222 ACS NSQIP hospitals. Surgery 2010; 148(4):625-35.

Jane Garbutt, Jane MBCh, Soper Nathaniel j, Shannon, William D, Botero Anna,et al. Meta analysis of Randomized controlled trials comprising Laparoscopic and open appendectomy. Surgical laparoscopy and endoscopy 1999; 9(1): 17-26.

Kamal M, Qureshi KH. Laparoscopic versus open appendectomy. Pak J Med Scein: 42: 23 - 26.

Kathouda N, Mason RJ, Towfigh S, GeyorgyannA, Essani R. Laparocopic versus open appendectomy: a prospective randomized double blind study. Ann Surg 2005; 242:439-448.

Konstadoulakis MM, Gomatos IP, Antonakis PT, Manouras A, Albanopoulas K, Nikiteas N, Leandros E,Bramis J. Two-trocar Laparoscopic assisted appendectomy versus conventional laparoscopic appendectomy in patients with acute appendicitis. J laparoendosc adv surg tech 2006; 16:27-32.

Koontz CS, Smith LA, Burkholder HC,Higdon K, Aderhold R, Carr M. Video assisted trans-umbilical appendectomy in children. J Pediatr Surg2006; 41:710-712.

Kehagias I, Karamanakos SN, Panagiotopoulos S, Panagopoulos K, Kalfarentzos F.Laparoscopic versus open appendectomy. Which way to go? World J Gastroenterol 2008; 14:4909-4914.

Lee SL, Yaqhoubian A, Kaji A. Laparoscopic versus open appendectomy in children: Outcomes comparison based on age, sex and perforation status.. Arch Surg 2011 [Epub ahead of print].

Malik AM, Talpur AH, Laghari AA. Video-assisted laparoscopic extra-corporeal appendectomy versus open appendectomy. J Laparoendosc Adv Surg Tech 2009; 19(3):355-9.

Mayer A, Preuss M, Roesler S, Lainka M, Omlor G. Transumbilical laparoscopic-assisted one-trocar appendectomy—TULAA—as an alternative operation method in the treatment of appendicitis.Zentralbl Chir 2004; 129(5): 391-5.

Ortega AE, Hunter JG, Peters JH, Swanstorm LL, Schirmer B. A prospective, randomized comparison of Laparoscopic appendectomy with open appendectomy. Laparoscopic appendectomy group. Am J Surg 1995; 169:20812?

Oannis Kehagias, stavros Nikolas Karanamanakos , Sypros Panagiotopoulos, Konstatinos Panagopoulos ,Fotis Kalfarentzos.Laparoscopic versus open appendectomy: which way to go? Worlf J Gastroenterol 2008; 14(31):4909-4914.

Olmi S, Magnone S, Bertolini A, Croce E. Laparoscopic versus open appendectomy in an acute appendicitis: a randomized prospective study. Surg Endosc. 2005; 19: 1193-95.

Pitfalls in laparoscopic appendectomy. J abdominal Emerg 2002; 22(6):889-894.

Rehman H, Rao AM, Ahmed. Single incision versus conventional multi-incision appendicectomy for suspected appendicitis. Cochrane database syst Rev 2011; 6; 7: CD009022.

Reiertsen O, Larsen S, Trondsen E,Edwin B, Faerden AE et al. Randomized controlled trial with sequential design of laparoscopic versus conventional appendicectomy.Br J Surg 1997;84: 842-7.

Roberts KE. True single-port appendectomy:first experience with the "Puppeteer technique". Surg endosc 2009;23(8):1825-30.

Shin EJ, Jeong GA, Jung JC, Cho GS, Lim CW et al. Transvaginal appendectomy. J Korean Soc Coloproctology 2010; 26(6): 429-32.

Santos BF, Hungness ES, Boller AM. Development of a feasible transrectal natural endocscopic surgery(NOTES) approach in a cadaveric appendectomy model: anterior is better. Surg Endosc 2011;.{Epub ahead of print}.

Saunders S, Lefering R, Neuqubauer EA. Laparoscopic versus open surgery for suspected appendicitis. Chochrane database sys rev 2002 ;(1): CD 00 1546.

Martin LC, Puente I, Sosa JL, Bassin A, Breslaw R, McKenney MG, E Ginzburg,Saleeman D. Open versus laparoscopic appendectomy. A prospective randomized comparison. Ann Surg 1995; 222(3):256-262.

Semm K. Endoscopic appendectomy. Endoscopy 1983; 15:59-64.

Suttie SA, Seth S, Driver CP, Mahomed AA. Outcome after intra-and -extra-corporeal laparoscopic appendectomy techniques. Surg Endosc 2004; 18(7): 1123-5.

Vipul D. Yagnik Jignesh B, rathod, Ajay G phatak. A retrospective study of two-port appendectomy and its comparison with open appendectomy and three port appendectomy. Saudi J Gastroenterol 2010; 16(4):268-271.

Valioulis I, Hameury F, Dahmani L, Levard G. Laparoscope-assisted appendectomy in children: the two trocar technique. Eur J pediatr Surg 2001; 11(6):391-4.

Wu SC, Wang YC, Fu CY, Chen RJ, Huang JC, Lu CW et al. Laparoscopic appendectomy provides better outcomes than open appendectomy in elderly patients. Am Surg 2011; 77(4):466-70.

Yano H, Murakami M, Nakano Y, Tone T, Ohnishi T, Iwazawa T et al. Laparoscopic treatment for perforated appendicitis with pelvic abscess. Digestive endoscopy 2004; 16:: 343-6.

Yoshikawa Seiichiro, Kidokoro Iba Tishiaki, Sugiysnma Kazuyushai, Fukunaga Tetsu et al.

2

Laparoscopic Management of Difficult Cholecystectomy

Mushtaq Chalkoo, Shahnawaz Ahangar, Ab Hamid Wani, Asim Laharwal, Umar Younus, Faud Sadiq Baqal and Sikender Iqbal
Department of Surgery, Government Medical College Srinagar, Kashmir, India

1. Introduction

Medicine is an ever changing art and needs to be shared with the progeny. Since the advent of laparoscopy, a new beginning started in the art of surgical craft. Many innovations and technical modifications are on the way for the satisfaction of the patient and the surgeon dealing with minimal access procedures. Laparoscopic cholecystectomy has revolutionized the whole globe and does not need any special mention. At the beginning surgeons would feel comfortable dealing with simple gallbladders but with the increase in expertise and introduction of newer armamentarium, difficult gallbladders are being subsequently dealt with. As of now, laparoscopic cholecystectomy can safely be declared as the gold standard for dealing with any kind of benign gallbladder disorder. However, before going to deal with the inflamed gallbladders; the skill of the surgeon, experience in laparoscopic techniques and thorough knowledge of risk factors are collectively important for a safe outcome. Even in the present era, the laparoscopic surgeon, amidst of such a substantial advance in laparoscopy, should have low threshold for conversion to open technique in case of difficulty. We strongly believe, from the experience we carry in dealing with these inflamed gallbladders, that every gallbladder is a book in itself which needs to be read time and again for a better and a safe outcome. Looking at the literature, the difficult thing to understand is to define the word 'difficult gallbladder.' However, we believe difficulty is a relative term and there are certain general principles that need to be followed before embarking on laparoscopic cholecystectomy. The aim of the operating surgeon should not only be giving the benefits of minimal access surgery but also avoiding the operative complications and lessen the postoperative morbidity.

The laparoscopic cholecystectomy is one of the common procedures performed globally so the errors are commonly reported. The beginners should start with the simple cases and the ideal patient would be one who is not obese, with no history of previous upper abdomen surgery, with a solitary stone in gallbladder and without features of cholecystitis. As the learning curve of the surgeon graphically increases, he can then deal with the difficult cases. We recommend the learning should be taken in a step ladder pattern. The patients having thick walled gallbladders, chronic cholecystitis, mucocele, inflamed Calot's triangle, previous upper abdomen surgeries, Mirrizi's, syndrome and obesity can be managed subsequently. Suture is future in laparoscopy. One needs to understand that difficult laparoscopy is a step ahead in this craft.

2. Risk factors

'Safety saves' is a golden principle in handling any surgical or operative procedure. A good navigator knows the trick of saving himself from the tides of misfortune. The risk is a part of surgical play and cannot be avoided but dealt with meticulously. The risk factors can be called the predictors of difficulty while performing the surgery. The clinical risk factors on history would be a stocky male patient, the reason of which is not clear till date, previous upper abdominal surgery, cirrhosis of liver, previous/present acute cholecystitis and/or acute pancreatitis, previous interventions like percutaneous drainage or cholecystostomy. A robust male patient is difficult to handle with respect to port creation, so is a very thin and lean patient. In the former the first port creation is difficult as lot of force is required for lifting the abdominal wall and then to to thrust in the first trocar while as in the latter, the possibility of intraabdominal injuries is common should the force required to put in the trocar not be guarded. The closely placed ports also pose a problem in the face of a simple gallbladder as it might result in sword fighting of the instruments.

Ultrasonography is a very important tool not only for diagnosing the gallbladder pathology but also predicting the difficulty during surgery. It is mandatory on the part of surgeon to know about the wall thickness, status of gallbladder (distended/contracted), solitary/multiple stones, cystic duct length and diameter, intrahepatic/extrahepatic gallbladder and above all the status of the common bile duct. The ultrasonic criteria for a difficult cholecystectomy can be categorized as under:

1. Thick walled gallbladder.
2. Contracted gallbladder
3. Gallbladder packed with stones.
4. A large calcified gallbladder
5. An acutely inflamed gallbladder, pericholecystic fluid collection and air in the gallbladder (emphysematous cholecystitis), xanthogranulomatous cholecystitis, acute gangrenous cholecystitis.
6. Left sided gallbladder.
7. Sessile gallbladder.

The risk factors that can arise while performing laparoscopic cholecystectomy are usually technical in nature. They can be enumerated as below

1. Difficult entry to the right hypochondrium owing to the adhesions.
2. Difficulty in exposure can also arise due to diseased gallbladder and Liver.
3. Acutely inflamed and tense gallbladder
4. Gallbladder packed with stones
5. Thick walled gallbladder
6. Fibrotic gallbladder
7. Gallbladder mass.
8. Abnormality can also arise due to anomalous anatomy of hepatobiliary system like situs inversus, malposition of the gallbladder, arterial anomalies and short cystic duct, a

huge stone impacted in the cystic duct, Hartmann's pouch adherent to the common hepatic duct and anomalous insertion of the cystic duct.

3. Safety measures

The difficulty encompasses a gamut of factors that arise from the patient, the surgical scene and the surgeon himself. The various safety measures in performing a safe laparoscopic cholecystectomy should not be undermined and left to the oblivion. The surgeon needs to give a due importance and weightage to all those techniques that will safeguard him for a smooth travel. One should resort to open laparoscopy in all those difficulties which make closed laparoscopy dangerous for the patient. The surgeon needs to be familiar with the angled scopes. Intraoperative cholangiography or laparoscopic ultrasound, if available, needs to be performed to identify the biliary anatomy and common duct stones. The adequate instrumentation is the key to a successful procedure. Toothed graspers are required to retract or grasp a thick walled gallbladder. The specialized needle drivers and holders are required. Hydrodissection is a boon to a safe surgery. One should not hesitate to create accessory ports for a speedy, safe and efficient outcome. One should be trained in suturing and knotting to encounter any difficulty that may arise while performing the procedure. Last, but not the least, one should always put in a drain in difficult circumstances. The proper positioning of patient adds ease to the surgeon. Partial or subtotal cholecystectomy sometimes proves to be the only alternative to the surgeon. One should not hesitate to leave the posterior wall intact in situations like fibrotic, intrahepatic and gangrenous gallbladders to avoid sinus opening and consequent bleeding.

4. Complications and technical difficulties

The various complications and the technical difficulties that we have come across from our experience of working with simple or difficult gallbladders for the last 10 years can be analyzed and discussed under the following categories

4.1 The problems related to the access to the operative site

4.1.1 Adhesions

It is a challenge to operate in the face of adhesions that could arise due to severe inflammatory conditions of gallbladder and as a result of any previous surgery. Owing to the operative scars in the lower abdomen designed for one or the other surgery, some amount of omental and bowel adhesions are very much common. In these situations it is better to avoid umbilicus as the initial site of veress needle insertion. It is better that one either resorts to open laparoscopy or else choose a safe site for the creation of pneumoperitoneum. One can even choose the site of the proposed epigastric port, slightly above the transpyloric plane in the midline. Some surgeons feel comfortable doing it in the left hypochondrium 2 cm below the subcostal margin in the midclavicular line with the due care to rule out spleenomegaly. One should not hesitate to use accessory ports to release the lower abdomen adhesions. The benefit of entering the abdomen this way avoids any inadvertent injury at the umbilicus as the port is put under visual guidance. The optical port can then be shifted from the epigastric to the umbilical site. One can also encounter small incisional hernias at the previous scar site which can then be repaired using polypropylene suture with or without mesh depending upon the size of the defect. Most of the previous surgeries done for appendix, ulcer disease or pancreas create a significant problem for the first port access. It is wise to resort to Hasson's technique or else go to the site that lies diagonal to the previous scar. The conversion rates to the tune of 25% have been reported in patients with extensive upper abdomen adhesions[2] .We do not recommend complete lysis of all the adhesions but would suggest only the obstructing adhesions to be lysed to clear the path for the camera port. All the bleeding points have to be controlled during adhesiolysis. These ports can be interchanged as camera and working trocars in order to get better exposure. We have an experience of going to laparoscopic cholecystectomy in patients with previous right upper paramedian incisions. We invariably would succeed to have a peep into the organ by a safe manipulation and rotation of the laparoscope to create a window through the adhesion. However, it may not be out of place to mention that the subsequent travel to the operative site for the camera assistant is a difficult job. The camera assistant needs to understand the negotiation of camera for a smooth and speedy outcome. Some surgeons use special trocars like visi-port or opti-view trocars to avoid any injury. But, they add cost to the procedure. Many studies have shown that the incidence of hollow viscus injury following open access for pneumoperitoneum and closed veress needle technique are the same.[3]

Inflammatory adhesions are very common due to acute cholecystitis or acute pancreatitis; but luckily they are usually flimsy and can easily be dealt with the suction nozzle. However, if the adhesions are dense, one should resort to the careful sharp dissection and control the diffuse self limiting oozes either with mild electrocautery or with a gauze piece. The predictors of dense adhesions in the subhepatic space from our experience can be grouped as under:-

1. Peptic ulcer surgery.
2. Right hemicolectomy.
3. Previous gastric surgery.
4. Hydatid cyst of liver.
5. Pancreaticodudenectomy.
6. Liver abscess surgery.

It is recommended, however, in face of dense adhesions, one can resort to additional ports, retrograde fundus-first technique or even modified cholecystectomy.

4.1.2 Incisional hernias

During laparoscopic cholecystectomy a surgeon can also deal with any concomitant hernias due to previous scars. However, one needs to understand and follow the principles of hernia repair. The problem of hernia is dealt with according to the site and size of the defect. The placement of mesh has to be avoided for small defects and in acute inflammatory or infective cases. The small hernias in and around umbilicus can usually be managed laparoscopically. We have a good experience of dealing with cholecystectomy and concomitant epigastric hernias laparoscopically in a single stage.

4.1.3 Morbid obesity

Obesity is associated with increased incidence of gallstone disease and it may also pose a problem of access. The patients who are morbidly obese are at risk of anesthetic and postoperative complications. The surgery in these patients is associated with a high incidence of pulmonary and thrombotic complications.[4] Pneumoperitoneum and steep

Trendelenberg position augment the risk of deep vein thrombosis. Obesity poses a difficulty for the beginners so far as the insertion of veress needle and first trocar is concerned. Calot's triangle is usually loaded with thick fat hence the identification of cystic duct and artery should be done carefully. Precautions that avoid any untoward event while operating on a patient with abdominal obesity are as follows:-

1. Adequate padding of the pressure points should be done. Lanz transumblical veress needle insertion technique may be applied. Two Lanz tissue holding forceps can be used to lift the umbilicus and with adequate muscle relaxation the surgeon can safely go into the abdomen perpendicular to the umbilicus after making a small incision. One should take proper care not to injure the skin at the site while lifting or holding the umbilicus. The surgeon needs to have a control on the thrust on insertion of Veress needle and the direction of the needle should be towards the pubic symphysis.
2. Sometimes the trocar length is a problem of concern for access. However, we have never used other than conventional trocars. The problem lies in the insertion of trocar. The amount of tension required to introduce trocar in abdominally obese patient is also a matter of concern. Most of the times the trocar might go into the parities and not into the abdominal cavity as such. Additionally, the trocar may go in an oblique fashion which creates difficulty in dissection for the surgeon.
3. Sometimes a thick fat laden falciform ligament creates a problem for the epigastric port. In difficult situations one can use a percutaneous silk stitch to lift it up.
4. The fat laden Calot's triangle sometimes obscures the anatomy. The dissection might sometimes cause torrential bleed from cystic artery if left unidentified. One can put a gauze piece and pack the area, relax for a minute and then proceed. The other way round is to get the fundus of gallbladder to the Calot's triangle and compress the area.
5. Sometimes the left lobe of the liver is enlarged and obscures the operating field. Left lateral tilting with placement of a sandbag behind the right costal margin moves it away from the field of surgery. However, from our working experience in such troubled matters we have learnt that the surgeon needs to be tricky to use his epigastric working port as a retractor as well as a dissector.

4.2 Technical difficulties that arise during cholecystectomy

A good navigator before embarking on his job should know his domain for a successful and smooth outcome. The technical difficulties that can arise while performing Laparoscopic cholecystectomy are varied in number. It is not possible to describe them in detail. Nevertheless, few of them do need a mention as under:-

4.2.1 Hidden gallbladder

Sometimes when the endoscope moves in, the surgeon doing diagnostic laparoscopy cannot find the gallbladder due to extensive adhesions. These adhesions between the inferior surface of the liver and the posterior parietal peritoneum together with hepatic flexure of colon and the omentum collectively seem to bury the gallbladder behind them. The duodenum may be adherent to the infundibulum. There may be even a fistulous communication between gallbladder and stomach or duodenum. The crux of the technique lies in moving in with suction nozzle and hydrodissection. The electrocautery should be carefully used. The surgeon needs to resort to careful sharp and blunt dissection. The fistulous communication needs to be looked for and if present should be repaired by intracorporeal suturing. If the gallbladder is hugely distended and tense, an initial decompression may ease the surgeon. However, we strongly recommend that mildly distended gallbladders should not be decompressed as the surgical planes become difficult to negotiate for the surgeon with the instruments. If the gallbladder is too thick and rigid, it is difficult for the surgeon to hold the gallbladder with his left hand and may further increase the difficulty. One can use toothed grasper to hold thickened gallbladder. Small and fibrotic gallbladders also add frustration to the surgeon and one needs to be patient to handle them safely.

4.2.2 Difficult retraction

The thick walled gallbladder is a problem for the assistant to hold and retract. The wall thickness beyond 4mm is a predictor of difficult retraction. Specialized toothed graspers with long and wide mouth can facilitate laparoscopic cholecystectomy. Similar maneuvers are also helpful in contracted gallbladder and gallbladders packed with stones. Long gallbladders, usually comma shaped, also pose a problem in retraction.

4.2.3 Bleeding

Bleeding is inherent to any surgical procedure. However, managing it intraoperatively is sometimes challenging for the surgeon. From our experience of 1000 laparoscopic cholecystectomies we have learnt that bleeding in no way should be considered an immediate reason for conversion. However, in rare circumstances, one should not hesitate to convert on account of profuse bleeding should the life of the patient be in jeopardy. During surgery bleeding may occur from injury to cystic artery or right hepatic artery. The bleeding from Calot's vascular arcade is usually mild and self limited which can be controlled by initial compression, clearing the field by suction nozzle followed by application of a clip, ligature or rarely electrocautery. The golden principle in laparoscopy look, hook and cook should always be kept in mind. Bleeding from cystic artery is sometimes profuse. Herein lies the test of patience of the surgeon. One should not panic and apply clips without having adequate vision. The cranial traction from the fundus of the gallbladder is released and the infundibulum is used to compress the bleeder. A gauze piece can also help in this situation. Most often bleeding stops due to spasm of the vessel. If bleeding is persistent one should be ready with the suction cannula to suck out the blood clots and with the left hand grasper, grasp the bleeding vessel. Meanwhile, after the area is clean, the clips are applied to the bleeder. Sometimes there is injury to the right hepatic artery which can be clipped if the liver is normal and there is no portal vein thrombosis. Bleeding can also arise from gallbladder bed which is usually diffuse ooze and can be controlled with an electrocautery (figure1). We have found that gel foams do not help much where as surgicel (oxydized cellulose polymer) is most effective in controlling bleeding from the liver bed. We also advocate packing of liver bed in case of opening up of a sinus with surgicel on top of which a wet-gauze should be placed and compressed by right hand forceps. Then the counter pressure should be maintained by the left hand forceps on the liver. This bimanual compression should be maintained continuously by watch for a period of 5 minutes (figure 2). We strongly believe that any kind of sinus bleed dealt in this way can be handled and conversion to open approach avoided to a great extent.

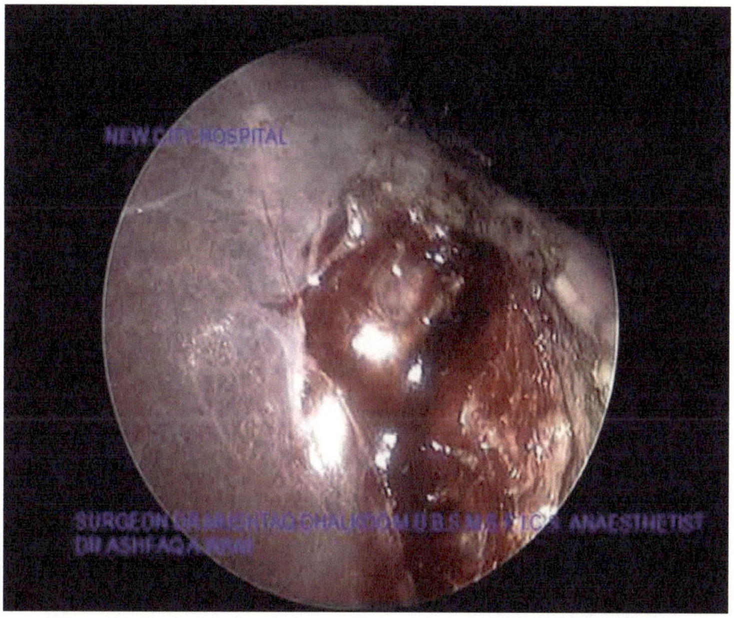

Fig. 1. Showing bleeding from one of the opened up sinues in the liver bed

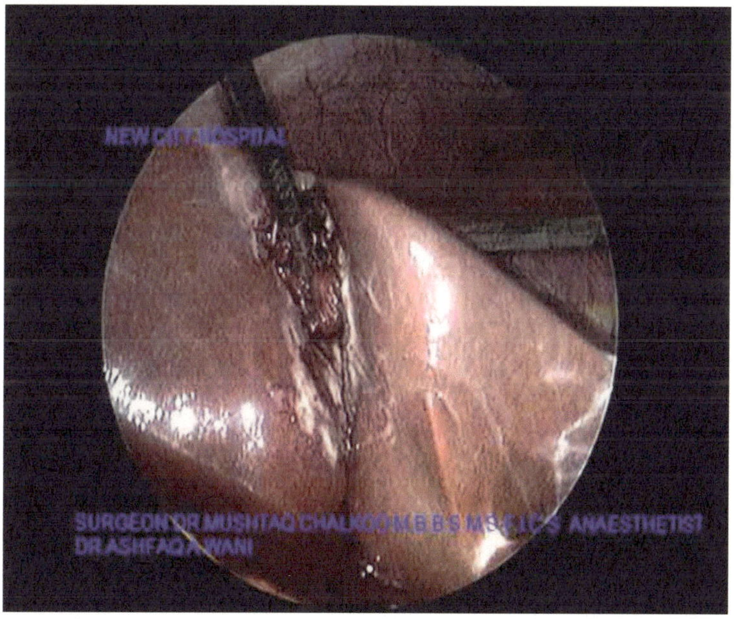

Fig. 2. Showing the application of pressure and counterpressure over a gauze.

4.2.4 Ductal injury

For a surgeon operating on the gallbladder, common bile duct needs to be safeguarded. Utmost care needs to be exercised to avoid ductal injury, whether a surgeon adopts open or laparoscopic approach to gallbladder. Ductal injuries do not only add morbidity to the patient but can even at times prove to be fatal. If the injury is recognized intraoperatively and treated immediately, the patient may do well. In our series of 1000 cholecystectomies done by laparoscopic approach fortunately we never encountered one. Nevertheless, two of our patients presented either with a bilioma (8th - 10th postoperative day) or biliary peritonitis (5th-7th postoperative day). Both of these were managed by re-laparoscopy wherein clearing the bile from the peritoneal cavity and putting in a wide bore 28F tube drain was done. One of these had a persistent leak through the drain till 35th postoperative day. The patient was later on subjected to ERCP and a biliary stent was put in which was then removed in the third month. Small biliomas in the Morrison's pouch or suprahepatic space can also be drained by percutaneous ultrasound guided technique. The ductal injury is a catastrophe that can result and hepaticojejunostomy can prove to be the only alternative for the operating surgeon. Sometimes accessory duct of Luscka is a cause for bilioma that a surgeon might not have recognized and dealt with in the initial go. In such a circumstance, re-laparoscopy with identification of accessory duct and clipping is recommended. If there is any bile leak which lasts beyond 5th postoperative day, distal block either with a stone or stenosis is likely. Our policy is to do ERCP and sphincterotomy with the extraction of the stone and stenting. In all such cases it takes just 24 hours for the leak to stop.

4.2.5 Malposition of the gallbladder

Sometimes the site of gallbladder other than the routine poses a challenge for the surgeon to operate. In dealing with such an exigency, many surgeons have come up with their own innovations with a view to facilitate and ease dissection. In situs inversus patients the surgeon stands in between the legs and the ports are placed mirror images of the routine ports (figure 3, 4). Here the epigastric is 5mm in size and the left subcostal port can be a 10 mm for the right hander's to facilitate clip application. The same arrangement of ports can be used in cases of left lobe gallbladder.

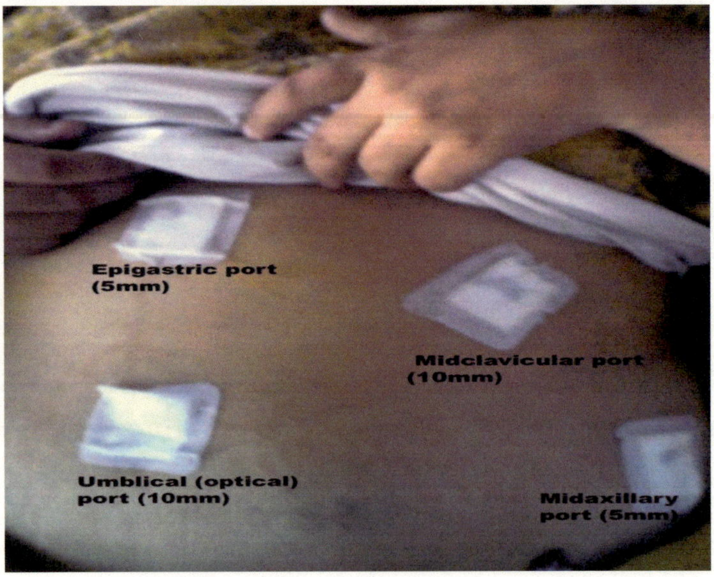

Fig. 3. Showing mirror image ports in Situs Inversus

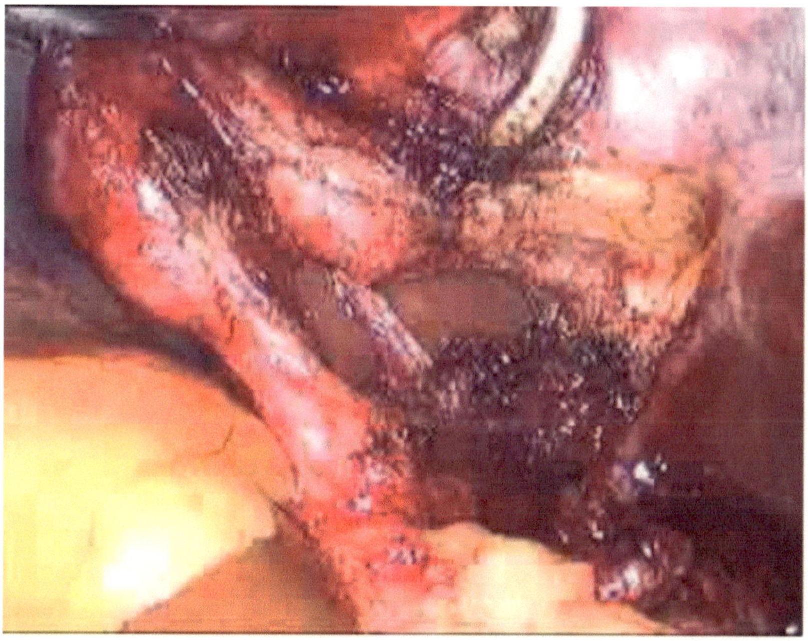

Fig. 4. Showing Critical view of safety in a situs inversus case

4.3 The problems related to the concomitant disease of gallbladder and nearby viscera

The gallbladder surgery has taken repute of many surgeons even at the distal end of their careers. A wise surgeon is one who thinks that the gallbladder, he operates on is his first one, amidst of huge experience he may carry in dealing with this organ. The difficulty while operating on an inflamed gallbladder cannot be defined. However, one needs to dissect safely to ease down the procedure. There are many problems and diseases of gallbladder that pose technical difficulties for the surgeon to remove this organ. One cannot generalize the principles for handling difficult gallbladders as each one of them poses a peculiar problem during dissection. The ones that need a mention herein are as follows:-

4.3.1 Impacted stone, hydrops, empyema, early Mirrizi's of gallbladder

In a situation where a huge stone is impacted in the neck of the gallbladder with resultant hydrops or empyema, the easy way out to handle such a gallbladder is to aspirate it after opening the fundus with a hot hook to perform suction irrigation (figure 5). One can make an incision on the neck of the gallbladder approximately 2-3 cm above the junction of cystic duct and the neck. This incision should be generous enough to allow for the exteriorization of the stone like an enucleation of the mass (figure 6). We have usually found that in such cases the cystic duct is either small or absent. In these big stones impacted at the neck or pouch, technical problem lies in holding the pouch by the left hand and consequent addition to the fatigue of the surgeon (figure 7).

Mirrizi's syndrome needs a mention. This syndrome was first described in 1948 by P.L. Mirrizi. He talked about an unusual complication of gallstones impacted either in the cystic duct or Hartmann's pouch and causing compression on the common hepatic duct to produce obstructive jaundice. The cause of jaundice is quite obvious either due to compression of the stone on the main duct or by a fistulous communication between Hartmann's pouch and the common hepatic duct. It occurs in 0.1 - 1.4% of all patients undergoing cholecystectomy. The clinical presentation is history of recurrent cholangitis, jaundice, right upper quadrant pain and abnormal liver function tests. Sometimes it may present as pancreatitis or acute cholecystitis. The presence of malignancy has to be excluded by computed tomography scan. It is wise to perform ERCP to study the ductal system before performing cholecystectomy in these patients. The laparoscopic management of Mirrizi's syndrome, once considered as a contraindication, can now be easily dealt with by an experienced laparoscopic surgeon confident in intracorporeal suturing and knotting. No doubt, it is a surgical challenge as the gallbladder is contracted and the visualization of biliary anatomy is poor due to extensive adhesions. The common bile duct may be mistaken for cystic duct and the chances of ductal injuries are more. Lastly, if the fistulous communication is not recognized, biliary peritonitis may occur.

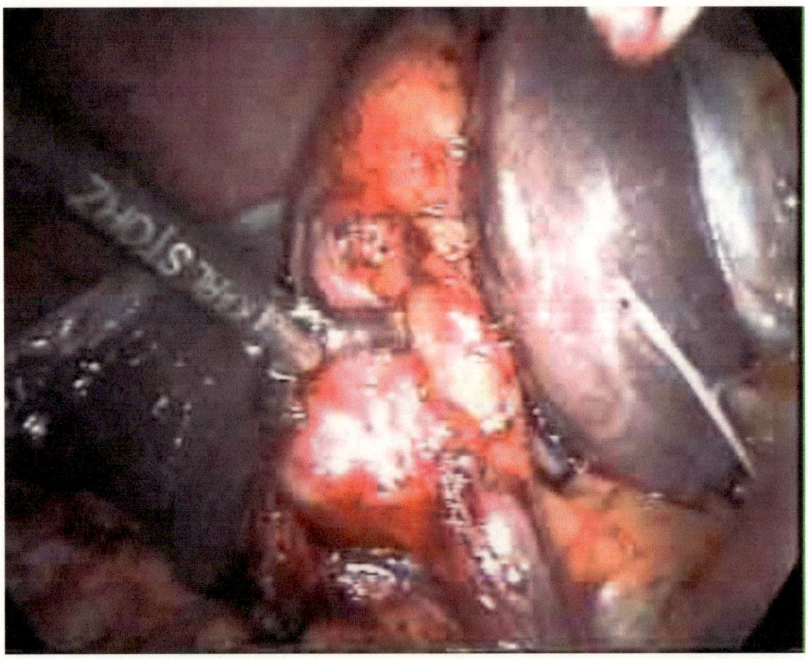

Fig. 5. Stone impacted at Hartmann's pouch.

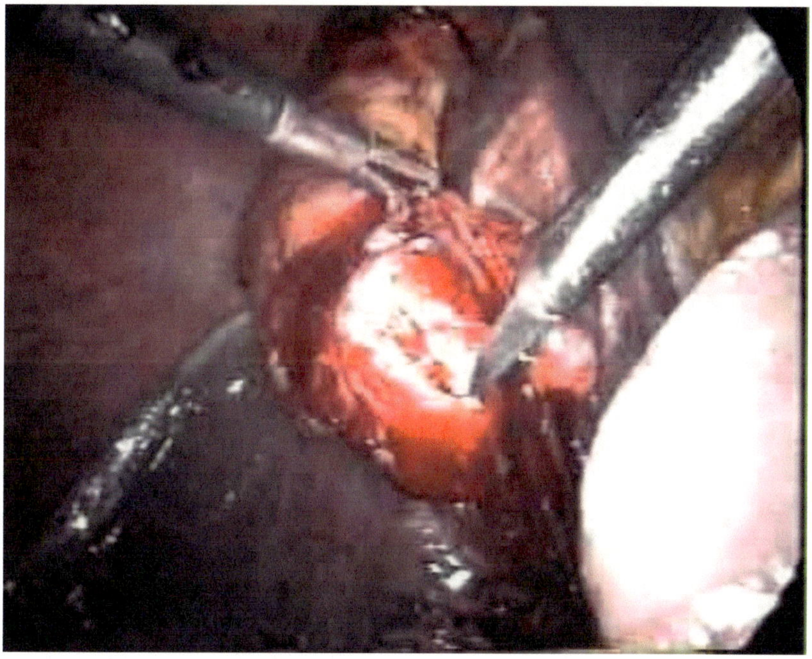

Fig. 6. Infundibulotomy done to remove the impacted stone.

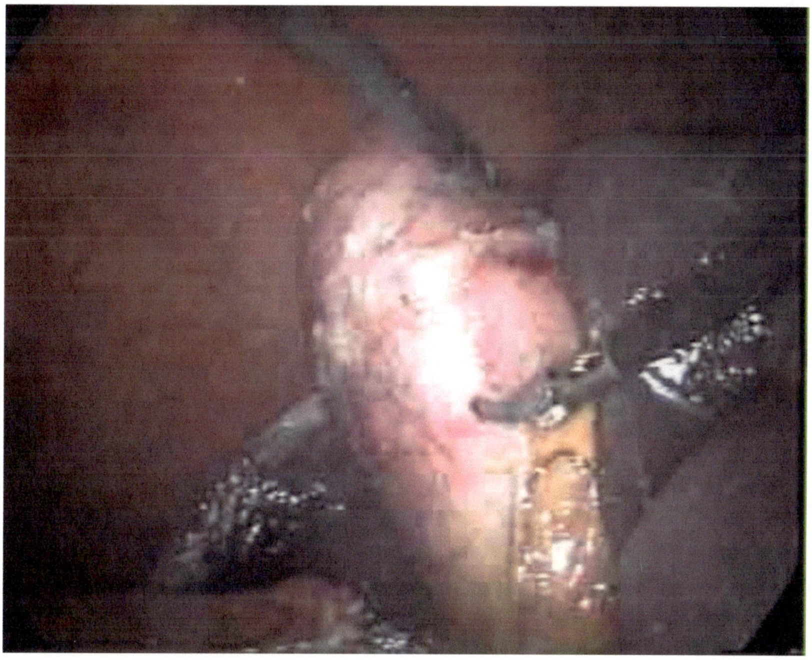

Fig. 7. Hydrops of the gallbladder

4.3.2 Acute gangrenous cholecystitis

Operating on acute cholecystitis should always be under taken by an experienced surgeon. One day or the other, one may come across an acute gangrenous cholecystitis (figure 8). One should remove all the inflammatory adhesions from the fundus of the gallbladder. It is safe to proceed with high pressure hydro-irrigation applied through a suction cannula in order to open up planes which are then further dissected using a grasper and scissors with electrocautery; staying away from the duodenum at all the times. Most of the surgeons might not go to dissect till the common bile duct is visible. They strongly feel that the dissection should be limited to the neck of the gallbladder. Even after the removal of the gallbladder, one may encounter a profuse continuous bleed from the liver bed possibly due to opening up of one of the sinuses as the planes are not clear. We usually use 2x2 cm gauze piece and a surgicel is left over the sinus for a period of five minutes to curtail the crisis. The spilt stones are usually a problem in handling such gallbladders. We recommend using a sterile endobag, if available, to remove the specimen and the stones together. After removal of the specimen, the port tract should be irrigated thoroughly.

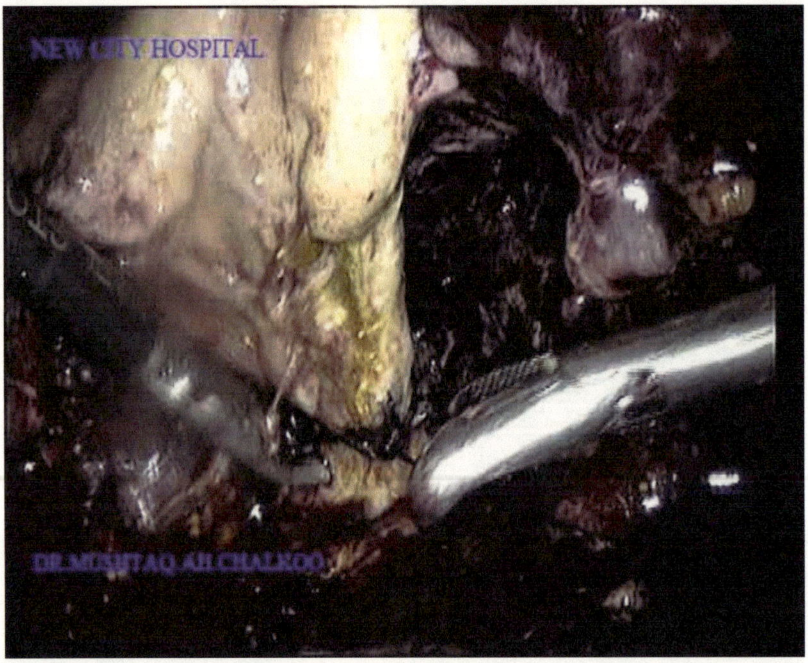

Fig. 8. Acute gangrenous cholecystitis.

4.3.3 Chronic cholecystitis

Handling a case of chronic cholecystitis is not easy too. The scleroatrophic cholecystitis is a challenge for the surgeon owing to a totally contracted, fibrosed and densely covered gallbladder with adhesions. The anatomical identification of structures is difficult. The initial fundus grasping is difficult. It is mandatory that fundus be released off the adhesions carefully. The loss of tissue planes is a problem in these cases because of repeated attacks of acute inflammation. The gallbladder is sometimes filled with stones or is a stone in itself and the retraction becomes difficult. There are more chances of injury to the common bile duct in handling this eventuality. One needs to be tricky to handle such a situation. The surgeon needs to have first glimpse of the gallbladder by releasing the adhesions. Additional port placement may help in this case. The retrograde technique may be then performed but should be done carefully. Intraoperative cholangiography may be done, if possible. The cystic duct is usually thick walled and difficult to occlude by clips. One should either use an endoloop or transfix the cystic duct after milking the duct towards the gallbladder to displace any stone, if present.

4.3.4 Cholecystoenteric fistula

This is an incidental finding during laparoscopic cholecystectomy and can account for 0.5-7% cases done laparoscopically for biliary disease (figure 9).[6] The diagnosis is suspected by noting the presence of air in the biliary tree associated with contracted gallbladder. The conditions where air is present within the biliary tree are infections by gas forming organisms, incompetent sphincter of Oddi, congenital anomalies, ERCP with sphincterotomy. Cholecystoduodenal, cholecystogastric and cholecystocolic are the common internal biliary fistulae. The common symptoms are pain, fever, diarrhea and jaundice. The most common cause for internal biliary fistulae is gallstones (90%) whereas; peptic ulcer, malignancy and trauma account for the rest 10% of the cases. Ultrasonography is useful and CT scan may show contracted, thick walled gallbladder with stones, pneumobilia and duodenal thickening. ERCP may localize the fistulous tract. Barium meal, enema and colonoscopy may be useful in the diagnosis.

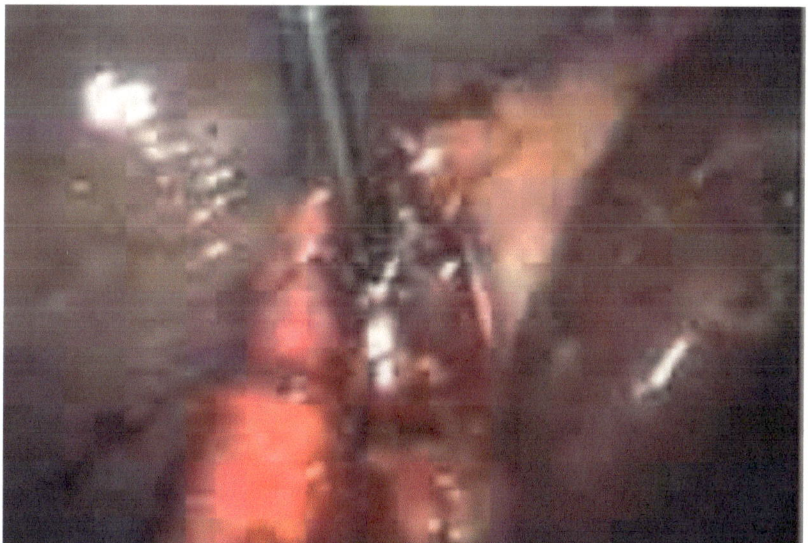

Fig. 9. Cholecystoenteric fistula.

4.3.5 Disorders of liver

It is a challenge for the surgeon to perform laparoscopic cholecystectomy in a patient with hepatic disorders especially cirrhosis. In near past this used to be considered a relative contraindication for the procedure as the mortality following cholecystectomy is 20 times more in cirrhotic than in non cirrhotic livers due to uncontrolled bleeding during surgery and deterioration of hepatic function in the postoperative period. With the passage of time, laparoscopic approach has now become the preferred procedure for symptomatic cholelithiasis in cirrhosis of liver in most of the hospitals. The reasons being that laparoscopy has an advantage of less blood loss, shorter operative time and a shorter length of hospitalization over the open approach. The liver function should be optimized before embarking on this procedure. The technical problems for the surgeon operating in the face of cirrhosis of liver are the adhesions with increased neovascularity, the problem of traction of liver, inadequate exposure of hilum, gallbladder bed with high risk of bleeding.

The periumblical collaterals might be a source of bleeding during initial trocar insertion. It is wise to use infraumblical route for Veress needle insertion. In case of portal hypertension the surgeon should alert himself and resort to minimum adhesiolysis. If possible, harmonic scalpel is effective in the process of adhesiolysis. If it is not available either bipolar cautery or clipping of the tortuous veins is highly recommended.

Retraction of liver may pose a problem to the surgeon as a result of hard fibrosis and contraction.

In situations where hilum cannot be exposed as a result of inadequate cranial traction on gallbladder the reasonable exposure should be obtained by lifting the body of the gallbladder instead of the fundus.

At times, the separation of posterior wall of the gallbladder from the liver bed is difficult or dangerous. In such circumstances, laparoscopic subtotal cholecystectomy or modified cholecystectomy is a sigh of relief to the surgeon.[5] Herein, we leave the posterior wall of the gallbladder intact with the liver and the mucosa is removed either by mucosectomy or by electrofulgration.

For a safe outcome, we recommend that for laparoscopic cholecystectomy in a patient of cirrhosis of liver, the hepatic dysfunction needs to be addressed first. Harmonic scalpel is extremely useful compared to monopolar electrocautery. Bleeding from the gallbladder bed can be treated by argon plasma coagulation, if available or using surgicel as a packing material in bleeding sinuses of the liver. Lastly, cholecystostomy should not be ignored in situations where cholecystectomy is dangerous.

4.3.6 Biliary pancreatitis

This is one of the difficult situations a surgeon can encounter in dealing with gallstone disease. Patients may also harbor a common duct stone. The cholecystectomy should be performed in the recovery phase which is around 10-60 days.[4] Any stone in the common bile duct detected by intraoperative cholangiogram or laparoscopic ultrasound can be managed simultaneously. In situations like progressive biliary obstructions, non responding cholangitis and drug resistant pancreatitis with a stone in the distal common bile duct, one should go for MRCP followed by ERCP. The technical problems in biliary pancreatitis for the surgeon is extensive adhesions, highly edematous cystic pedicle and hepatoduodenal ligament, presence of ascitic fluid, pseudocystic pancreas in retrogastric position. In situations like these, interval cholecystectomy is advised.

We recommend an early cholecystectomy in a patient with multiple small stones to avoid recurrent bouts of pancreatitis. It may also be useful to categorize the patients into mild and severe degrees for directing appropriate management. Currently the best method to assess the severity of acute pancreatitis is contrast enhanced computed tomography scan. It is understood that biliary pancreatitis is due to a transient block of the ampulla of Vater by a migrating stone from gallbladder. It is a proven fact that the stone passes to the duodenum in majority of cases within hours of the onset of pancreatitis. If the acute process is increasing and reveals persistent obstruction, ERCP should be performed. Endoscopic sphincterotomy and extraction of the stone allows the acute pancreatitis to settle down. In mild pancreatitis laparoscopic cholecystectomy can be performed safely at the initial admission within first week depending on the condition of the patient. It is wise also to have an intraoperative cholangiogram as the risk of concurrent common bile duct stones is 14-20% associated with biliary pancreatitis. It may not be out of place to mention the value of MRCP and ERCP in severe cases. Currently an endoscopist and a laparoscopist work together to manage the problem of common bile duct stones as laparoscopic exploration of common bile duct is considered a high risk procedure in the phase of acute biliary pancreatitis.

4.3.7 Porcelain gallbladder

Here the gallbladder wall is deposited with calcium. The prevalence in cholecystectomy specimens ranges from 0.06 - 0.08%. [7,8] It usually occurs in elderly persons with gallstones who are predominantly females. X-ray abdomen may show a calcified lesion in the right upper quadrant. Ultrasonography and CT scan rule out the presence of an associated carcinoma. It increases the risk of carcinoma gallbladder by 12.5 - 60%.[4] However, it is still debatable. The removal of gallbladder is the treatment of choice. It is a technically demanding surgery. However, adequate care should be taken to prevent dissemination of malignant cells in the abdominal cavity and port site, if present. The specimen bags are essential for gallbladder retrieval.

4.3.8 Carcinoma gallbladder

Carcinoma of the gallbladder is estimated to be present in 1% of cholecystectomy specimens. It is the most common malignancy of the biliary tract. It is usually common in females.[4] 85% of the cases are associated with the gallstones. It is recommended by the current medicine that a gallbladder polyp of more than 10mm size should undergo cholecystectomy.[4] The smaller polyps should be followed up at 6 monthly periods and any increase in size is an indication for cholecystectomy. The incidental gallbladder carcinoma is diagnosed postoperatively by the histopathological examination of the specimen removed for the gallstone disease. During surgery it is advocated that the surgeon should avoid inadvertent disruption of gallbladder to avoid spillage of malignant cells into the peritoneal cavity and the gallbladder should be removed in an endobag to avoid portal metastasis.

5. Conclusion

We strongly believe that every difficulty has a loop-hole that needs to be exploited to ease down the procedure. Before embarking on difficult cholecystectomies, a surgeon needs to be trained in all the technical aspects of laparoscopy. A due care should be given to suturing skills. Every gallbladder should be dealt with as if the surgeon, regardless of the experience, is operating on the first gallbladder. The general principles in laparoscopy and the critical view of safety should always be born in mind. The theatre staff especially the cameraman should be properly trained. The instruments should be quite friendly and a surplus of them should be available. The surgeon should have had a good amount of experience with simple gallbladders before handling the difficult ones. With the advent of gratifying improvements in the imaging technology, instrumentation and innovative techniques, the difficult gallbladders now fall in the domain of simple surgeries. However, the intrinsic error in the surgical technique cannot be avoided and whenever it comes onto that, open approach should always be given a weightage.

6. References

[1] Mushtaq Chalkoo.,2009. Laparoscopic Cholecystectomy in a Mucocele of Gallbladderwith a Phrygian Cap- A Case Report,[online]. Available at: web address: http://www.google.co.in/search?sourceid=chrome&ie=UTF8&q=phyicians+academy+online+mushtaq+chalkoo

[2] Jorgensen JO, Hunt DR. Laparoscopic cholecystectomy. A prospective analysis of the potential causes of failure. Surg Laparosc Endosc. 1993 Feb;3(1):49-53.

[3] Patel M, Smart D. Aust N Z J Surg. Laparoscopic cholecystectomy and previous abdominal surgery: a safe technique. 1996 May;66(5):309-11

[4] Palanivelu C., 2007. Art of laparoscopic surgery. Ist ed. New Delhi: Jaypee.

[5] K. Michalowski, P. C. Bornman, Professor J. E. J. Krige, P. J. Gallagher, J. Terblanche. Laparoscopic subtotal cholecystectomy in patients with complicated acute cholecystitis or fibrosis. Volume 85, Issue 7, pages 904–906, July 1998

[6] Nadu A, Gallili Y, Soffer D, Kluger Y. J Trauma. Disruption of cholecystoenteric fistula induced by minor blunt trauma. 1996 Nov;41(5):914-5.

[7] Puia IC, Vlad L, Iancu C, Al-Hajjar N, Pop F, Bălă O, Munteanu D. Chirurgia (Bucur). Laparoscopic cholecystectomy for porcelain gallbladder. 2005 Mar-Apr;100(2): 187-9.

[8] Polk HC Jr. carcinoma and the calcified gallbladder. Gastroenterology 1966;50: 582-5.

3

Laparoscopic Pancreatic Surgery

Jin-Young Jang
Department of Surgery, Seoul National University College of Medicine, Seoul, Korea

1. Introduction

Pancreatic surgery has higher morbidity and mortality than other forms of gastrointestinal tract surgery, due to associated problems like pancreatic fistula formation and loss of pancreatic function. Until recently laparoscopic surgery of the pancreas was limited to laparoscopic staging or to the evaluation of periampullary cancer for detecting small metastatic nodules or local invasion (Jang et al., 2007; Schachter et al., 2000). Advances in laparoscopic techniques and instrumentation have expanded the role of laparoscopic surgery to a degree that could not have been imagined such as Whipple's procedure (Gagner & Gentileschi, 2001).

Recent reports on laparoscopic surgery of the pancreas are encouraging and support the advantages of laparoscopy. We believe that well selected enucleation and laparoscopic distal pancreatectomy, with or without spleen preservation, are acceptable and recommendable for the treatment of benign or low grade malignant diseases of the pancreas. Moreover, surgeons and laparoscopic industries have developed new techniques and devices that increase convenience, ease, and safety of complicated laparoscopic surgeries, and these efforts will undoubtedly increase the role of laparoscopic or minimal invasive surgery for the treatment of pancreatic disease.

In this chapter, we will discuss the current status of the laparoscopic pancreatic surgery and the role of its associated procedures for the treatment of pancreatic disease.

2. Pancreatic resection

2.1 Distal pancreatectomy

Although laparoscopic pancreatic surgery is considered to be an advanced and demanding procedure, many surgeons have tried laparoscopic distal pancreatectomy due to its technical simplicity and its avoidance of the need for anastomosis as compared with other difficult pancreatectomy (Table 1) (Weber et al., 2009; Mabrut et al., 2005; Melotti et al., 2007; Vijan et al., 2010; Fernandez-Cruz et al., 2007; Røsok et al., 2010; DiNorcia et al., 2010; Jayaraman et al., 2010; Kooby et al., 2008; Song et al., 2011; Velanovich, 2006; Misawa et al., 2007; Teh et al., 2007; Kim et al., 2008; Matsumoto et al., 2008; Eom et al., 2008; Nakamura et al., 2009).

Most of reports demonstrate the feasibility of laparoscopic approach with acceptable morbidity (10~30%) and nearly no mortality.

Study	Cases	Multi-Instituti-onal	Mean Operative Time (min)	Mean Blood Loss (mL)	Length of Stay (day)	Conversion Rate (%)	Splenic Preservation (%)	Overall Morbidity (%)	Pancreatic Fistula Rate (%)	Mortality (%)
Weber, 2009	219	Y	219	245	2.6	10	34	39	23	0
Mabrut, 2005	96	Y	200[a] 195[b]	N/A	7	10	71	53	16	0
Melotti, 2007	58	Y	165	N/A	9	0	55	53	27.5	0
Vijan, 2010	100	N	214	171	6.1	4	25	34	17	3
Fernandez-Cruz, 2007	82	N	N/A	N/A	7	7	64	20	9	0
Rosok, 2010	117	N	185.5[a] 210[b]	200[a] 100[b]	5	7.5	32	16.5	10	N/A
DiNorcia, 2010	95	N	250	150	5	25.3	15.5	28.2	11.3	0
Jayaraman, 2010	107	N	193	150	5	30	21	20	15	0
Kooby, 2008	167	Y	230	357	5.9	13	31	40	11	0
Song, 2011	359	N	195	N/A	8	N/A	49.6	12	7	0

[a] With splenic preservation
[b] With splenectomy
N/A (Not Available Values)

Table 1. Recently published reports of laparoscopic distal pancreatectomy

Study	Cases		Mean Operative Time (min)		Mean Blood Loss (mL)		Splenic Preservation (%)		Length of Stay (day)		Overall Morbidity (%)		Pancreatic Fistula Rate (%)		Mortality (%)	
	LDP	ODP	LDP	ODP	LDP	ODP	LDP	ODP	LDP	ODP	LDP	ODP	LDP	ODP	LDP	ODP
Velanovich, 2006	15	15	N/A	N/A	N/A	N/A	0	0	5.0	8.0	20	27	13	13	0	0
Misawa, 2007	8	9	255	205	14	307	12.5	0	10.0	16.0	N/A	N/A	0	22	0	0
The, 2007	12	16	278	212	193	609	62	17	6.2	10.6	17	56	8	6	0	0
Kim, 2008	93	35	195	190	110	110	40.8	5.7	10	16	25	29	8.6	14.3	0	0
Matsumoto, 2008	14	19	291	213	247	400	7	N/A	12.9	23.8	N/A	N/A	0	110.5	0	0
Eom, 2008	31	62	218	195	N/A	N/A	42	N/A	11.5	13.5	36	24	9.7	6.5	0	0
Nakamura, 2009	21	16	308	282	249	714	35	31	10.0	25.8	0	19	0	12.5	0	0
Jayaraman, 2010	107	236	163	193	150	350	21	14	5	7	27	40	15	13	0	2
Kooby, 2008	142	200	230	216	357	588	30	12	5.9	9.0	40	57	11	18	0	1

Table 2. Comparisons of laparoscopic and Open distal pancreatectomy

According to several reports comparing the clinical results of laparoscopic surgery with open surgery, no statistical differences were found in terms of operation time, morbidity, or recurrence. However, mean length of hospital stay was shorter in the laparoscopic group than in the open surgery group (Table 2) (Vijan et al., 2010; Kooby et al., 2008; Velanovich, 2006; Misawa et al., 2007; Teh et al., 2007; Kim et al., 2008; Matsumoto et al., 2008; Eom et al., 2008; Nakamura et al., 2009).

We could conclude that laparoscopic distal pancreatectomy is a safe and feasible method equivalent to open distal pancreatectomy in terms of early and late outcome for benign and borderline lesions of pancreas such as pancreas cystic neoplasms and neuroendocrine tumors. Considering superior cosmetic results and early functional recovery, laparoscopic distal pancreatectomy could be treatment of choice in most of non-cancerous diseases located at pancreas body and tail.

The role of laparoscopic distal pancreatectomy for the treatment of pancreatic cancer remains controversial. Many pancreatic surgeons worry about the oncological safety of laparoscopic pancreatectomy in relation to surgical margin, retroperitoneal clearance, and retrieval of peripancreatic lymph node (Kubota, 2011; Kooby & Chu, 2010).

Several reports showed that laparoscopic distal pancreatectomy provided similar short- and long-term oncologic outcomes as compared with open surgery, with potentially shorter hospital stay even in pancreatic cancer. These results suggest that laparoscopic distal pancreatectomy is an acceptable approach for resection of pancreatic ductal adenocarcinoma (PDAC) of the left pancreas in selected patients (Kooby & Chu, 2010; Dulucq et al., 2005; Kooby et al., 2010).

Although the result of laparoscopic distal pancreatectomy for pancreatic cancer seems to be favorable in limited cases, we must wait for more long term results to reach a conclusion on oncological safety of laparoscopic resection for pancreatic cancer.

Spleen preservation and method of preservation are important issues of laparoscopic distal pancreatectomy, and surgeons showed diverse preferences for surgical method (Table 1). Spleen-preserving distal pancreatectomy was introduced by Mallet et al. in 1943 (Mallet & Vachon, 1943), and as knowledge of the immunologic role of spleen increased, efforts to conserve the organ have intensified (Robey et al., 1982; Yamaguchi et al., 2001).

According to the recently published data, 15~70% of distal pancreatectomies were performed preserving spleen (Table 1). Two techniques are employed during spleen-preserving operations. The first involves splenic artery and vein transection such that the left gastroepiploic vessels and short left gastric vessels will supply the spleen (Warshaw's technique) (Warshaw, 1997), whereas in the second the splenic artery and vein are preserved (Figure 1).

This second method demands more advanced instrumentation and skill in terms of dividing the transverse branches of splenic vessels and has a risk of left-sided portal hypertension if the splenic vein becomes occluded after surgery (Yoon et al., 2009).

Whereas Warshaw's technique is technically easy and requires shorter operative time (Kaneko et al., 2004; Mori et al., 2005), it may result in splenic infarction and splenic abscess formation due to insufficient blood flow to the spleen (Warshaw, 1997).

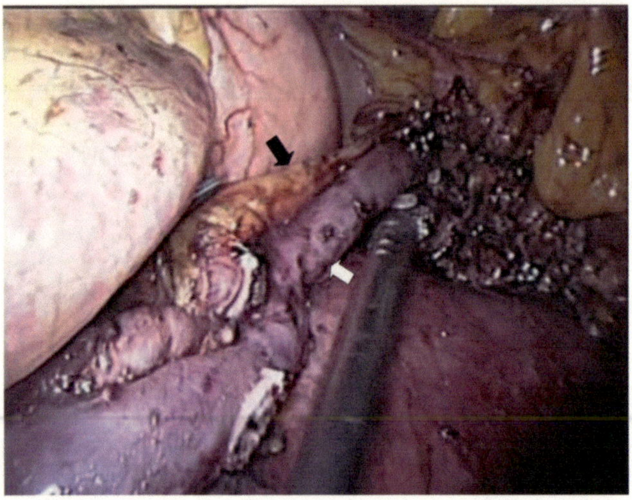

Black arrow: preserved splenic artery
White arrow: preserved splenic vein

Fig. 1. Laparoscopic spleen preserving distal pancreatectomy.

2.2 Pancreatoduodenectomy

Although laparoscopic pancreatoduodenectomy was introduced at 1994 by Dr. Gagner (Gagner & Pomp, 1994), this procedure is still technically challenging.

There have been limited case reports on laparoscopic pancreatoduodenectomy (Table 3) (Gagner & Pomp, 1997; Staudacher et al., 2005; Dulucq et al., 2006; Palanivelu et al., 2007; Pugliese et al., 2008; Cho et al., 2009; Kendrick & Cusati, 2010), and some surgeons advocate its safety and feasibility. However, lack of tactile sensation, difficulties in localizing lesions, and the anatomic complexity of peripancreatic organs to make laparoscopic pancreatoduodenectomy difficult (Cuschieri, 1996).

Even Dr. Gagner, the initiator of laparoscopic pancreatoduodenectomy, concluded that this procedure offers no advantage in terms of patient outcome and may be associated with increased morbidity (Gagner & Pomp, 1997). Nevertheless, laparoscopic experience has allowed some surgeons to claim promising results for laparoscopic pancreatoduodenectomy (Gagner & Pomp, 1997; Staudacher et al., 2005; Dulucq et al., 2006; Palanivelu et al., 2007; Pugliese et al., 2008; Cho et al., 2009; Kendrick & Cusati, 2010; Cuschieri, 1996).

However, laparoscopic pancreatoduodenectomy has many pitfalls. Pancreatoduodenectomy itself requires meticulous anastomosis to reduce morbidities associated with pancreatic leakage, and adequate dissection to remove diseased tissue including lymph nodes and nerve plexus. Small operative windows cannot highlight the merit of minimally invasive surgery in pancreatoduodenectomy because of the long operation time and high morbidity due to pancreato-enteric anastomosis.

On the other hand, it can be expected that technical advances, like robotic surgery (Makary, 2011; Horiguchi et al., 2011), will continue to make pancreatoduodenectomy by minimal invasive surgery more feasible and safe.

Study	Cases	Pathology	Conversion Rate (%)	Hand assist (%)	Operative Time (min)	Blood Loss (mL)	Length of Stay (day)	Overall Morbidity (%)	Pancreatic Fistula Rate (%)	Mortality (%)	Mean nodes procured	Positive margin for Malig. (%)
Gagner & Pomp, 1997	10	4 PDAC, 3 AMP, 2 pancreatitis, 1 CC	40	33	510	N/A	22.3	17	50	0	7(3-14)	0
Staudacher, 2005	7	2 PNET, 1 PDAC, 4 etc	43	100	416	325	12				26(16-47)	0
Dulucq, 2006	25	11 PDAC, 4 AMP, 2 DA, 1 PNET, 2 pancreatitis, 2 etc	12	41	287	107	16.2		32	4.5	18(N/A)	0
Palanivelu, 2007	42	24 AMP, 9 PDAC, 4 MCA, 3 CC, 2 pancreatitis	0	0	370	65	10.2	7.1	N/A	2.4	13(8-21)	0
Pugliese, 2008	19	6 PDAC, 4 AMP, 3 etc	32	54	461	180	18	23	37	0	12(4-22)	0
Cho, 2009	15	6 IPMN,3 IPMC, 2 PNET, 1 AMP, 1 PDAC, 2 etc	0	100	338	445	16.4	13	27	0	18.5(N/A)	0

AMP, ampullary adenocarcinoma/ampullary dysplastic adenoma; CC, cholangiocarcinoma; DA, duodenal adenocarcinoma; CA, mucinous cystadenocarcinoma;; N/A, not reported; PDAC, pancreatic ductal adenocarcinoma; PNET, pancreatic neuroendocrine tumor

Table 3. Published reports of laparoscopic pancreatoduodenectomy

2.3 Other miscellaneous pancreatectomy and palliative procedures

Enucleation is one of commonly conducted procedures of laparoscopic pancreatectomy. According to a review by Tagaya et al (Tagaya et al., 2003), laparoscopic enucleation has been used to treat relatively small benign or low grade malignancies, and tumors located on the surface of the pancreas remote from the pancreatic duct. Tumor location is an important factor for successful laparoscopic enucleation to avoid pancreatic duct injury, and some advocate that enucleation is a safe and simple procedure under laparoscopic ultrasonographic guidance (Matsumoto et al., 1999).

The enucleation offers the possibility of complete tumor removal without loss of pancreatic parenchyma, possible diabetes, and splenectomy in some endocrine tumor or pancreatic cystic neoplasm. However, enucleation seems to be a debatable procedure in patients with pancreas cystic tumors, and does not address the malignant potential of these tumors, and thus, should be used cautiously in selected cases to avoid inadequate safe surgical margins and rupture (Fernandez-Cruz et al., 2005). In addition, the incidence of pancreatic fistula after tumor enucleation has been reported to be 30% to 75%, which is relatively higher than that of conventional pancreatectomy (Pyke et al., 1992; Talamini et al., 1998; Iihara et al., 2001). Moreover, considerations of oncological and operational safety require that surgeons exercise caution when selecting indications for laparoscopic enucleation.

Some surgeons have developed more intricate procedures like laparoscopic central pancreatectomy and ventral pancreatectomy (Orsenigo et al., 2006; Kang et al., 2011; Giulianotti et al., 2010).

Laparoscopy may be used in a palliative context for locally advanced or metastatic pancreatic/periampullary cancers. Many patients with periampullary cancer have symptoms associated with biliary or gastric outlet obstruction, and traditionally these patients have been managed by open bypass surgery. Recently, minimally invasive laparoscopic approaches to gastric and biliary bypass have been successfully applied, and have been shown by non-randomized comparative studies to be safer and to be associated with reduced periods of hospitalization than open surgery (Schwarz & Beger, 2000; Bergamaschi et al., 1998; Rothlin et al., 1999; Rhodes et al., 1995).

Although endoscopic or radiologic procedures for palliative treatment have been enormously developed and have achieved early success rates for endoscopic stent which is comparable to those of surgery with reduced morbidity and hospital stays, the long-term results of endoscopic procedures are not as satisfactory (van den Bosch et al., 1994). Thus, randomized comparisons of laparoscopic biliary bypass and interventional biliary stents in unresectable periampullary cancer are needed.

3. Laparoscopic diagnosis/staging

Laparoscopic diagnosis and staging are controversial in patients with suspected pancreatic cancer. Its main role is to detect occult intra-abdominal metastatic disease, during the procedure any suspicious lesion can be biopsied and peritoneal cytology can also be obtained by instilling normal saline into the peritoneum (Michl et al., 2006; Merchant et al., 1999; Nieveen van Dijkum et al., 1999).

The yield of laparoscopy for the detection of metastatic disease, especially of small peritoneal lesions that have not been detected by imaging modalities, ranges from 15 to 46% (Jimenez et al., 2000; Menack et al., 2001; Minnard et al., 1998; Velasco et al., 1998; Liu & Traverso, 2005). Recent studies have shown lower yields for laparoscopy than for improved non invasive imaging modalities like multi detector CT. The yield of laparoscopy alone is clearly impaired by its inability to detect locally advanced or intra-parenchymal liver disease. To overcome this obvious limitation, laparoscopic ultrasound has been added to laparoscopic staging, and this leads to a marked increase in yield and accuracy (Dulucq et al., 2006). Studies comparing laparoscopy and laparoscopic ultrasound with radiological staging modalities have produced controversial results. However, several studies have found that laparoscopy and laparoscopic ultrasound are more accurate than contrast-enhanced CT at determining T stage (John et al., 1999; Doran et al., 2004).

In contrast, three large studies using contrast-enhanced multi-detector CT imaging as a baseline radiological investigation were unable to confirm this, and found yields as low as 10-15% and accuracies of 35-56% for laparoscopy (Nieveen van Dijkum et al., 2003; Brooks et al., 2002). Despite the use of a pre-operative staging algorithm including laparoscopic ultrasound, up to 20% of patients were still found to be unresectable at the time of laparotomy, mainly because of local invasion (Talamini et al., 1998). Moreover, as diagnostic yields have fallen, due to improvements in non-invasive imaging, the additional costs of laparoscopy have been called into question, particularly since it requires separate anesthesia. Thus, at present, laparoscopy has a limited role in the staging of peri-pancreatic malignancies (Michl et al., 2006).

4. Laparoscopic application to pancreatitis

The role of surgery in the management of acute pancreatitis is markedly being reduced because less invasive intervention and intensive medical care are evolving. Although some clinicians advocate a non surgical approach even in cases of infected necrotizing pancreatitis, due to the improved results of medical or interventional treatment (Chang et al., 2006), current indications for surgery in pancreatitis are infected necrotizing pancreatitis, an organizing pseudocyst, or related complications.

The treatment of infected necrosis has changed dramatically during the last few years, and a multimodality approach has emerged, where a combination of several techniques are used in a single patient, and the risks of intervention are weighed against the need for adequate sepsis control (Garden, 2005).

Minimally invasive surgery has consistently been shown to be associated with reduced inflammatory response activation than equivalent open surgery, and some evidence suggests that local sepsis and inflammatory response may also be lessened by minimally invasive surgery. It has been suggested that by minimizing the massive inflammatory injury associated with open pancreatic necrosectomy, a minimally invasive approach to the management of infected pancreatic necrosis may lessen the risk of multiple organ failure, and reduce respiratory and wound morbidity in necrotizing pancreatitis (Garden, 2005; Parekh, 2006).

The laparoscopic approach depends on the localization of pancreatic necrosis. The alternatives are an intraperitoneal approach, direct entry of the retroperitoneal space, and an intraperitoneal transgastric approach. Our group experienced three successful cases of laparoscopic necrosectomy using a multiple approach technique for necrotizing pancreatitis (Figure 2). The potential benefits of minimal invasive techniques are yet to be proven, because of a rarity of reports that deal with severely ill patients, and thus, the superiority or inferiority of laparoscopic over endoscopic or radiologic intervention must be proven by randomized prospective study.

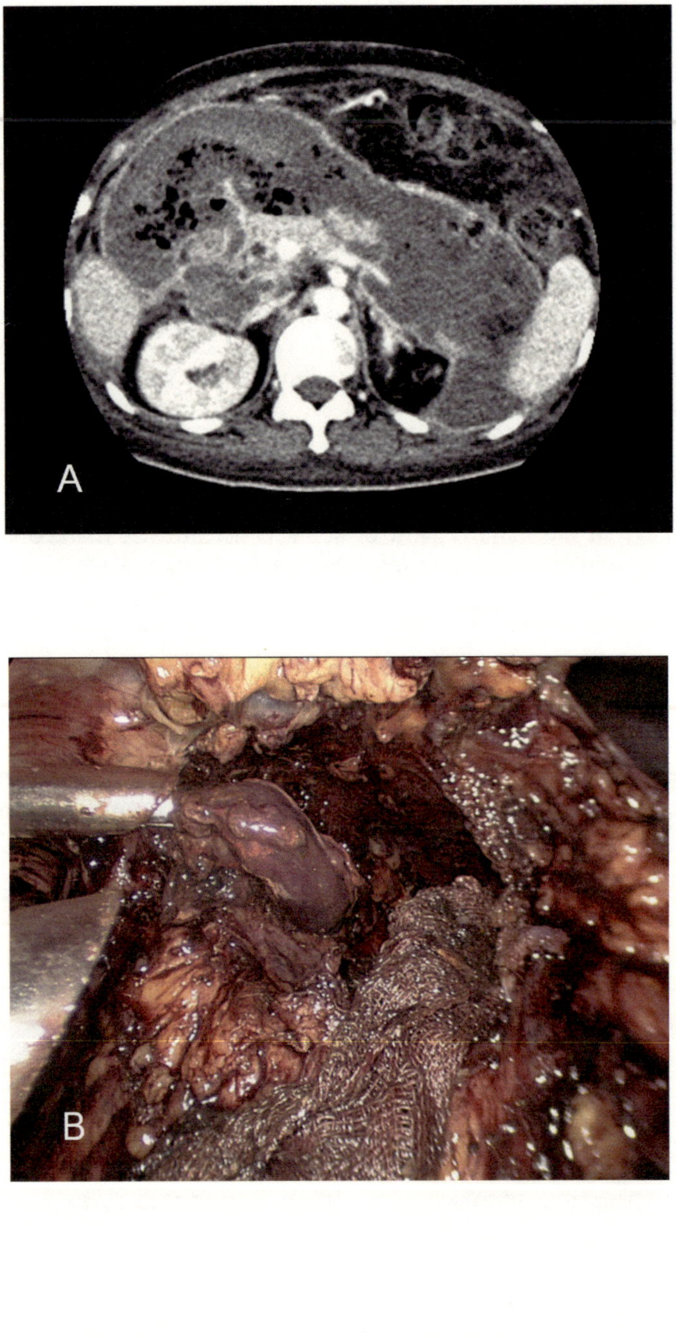

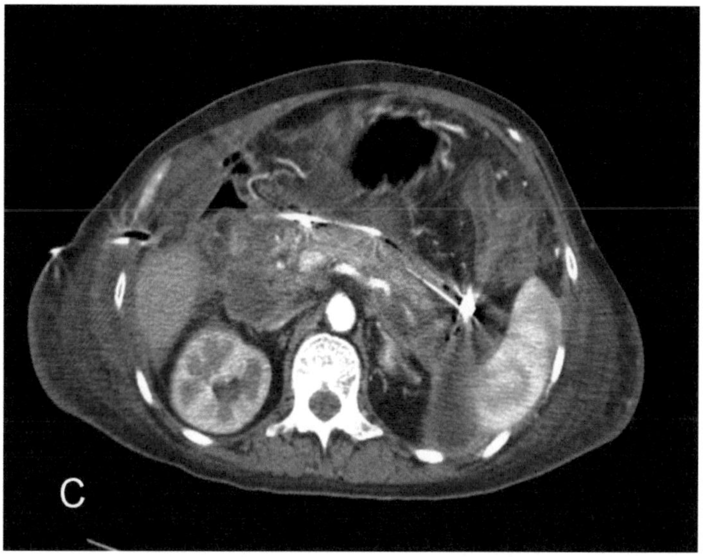

(A) CT shows severe necrosis around pancreas.
(B) Necrosis was laparoscopically approached and debrided using gauze and forceps.
(C) Postoperative CT shows marked decrease of necrotic area around pancreas.

Fig. 2. A 38 year old man, with severe necrotizing pancreatitis, was successfully managed by laparoscopic approach.

The management of pancreatic pseudocyst, complicated (acute or chronic) pancreatitis represents another important role of laparoscopy in pancreatitis. Pseudocysts complicate 5 10% of acute pancreatitis attacks and often arise as a result of disruption of the pancreatic duct in the presence of gland necrosis. Large (≥6cm diameter), persistent (≥6 weeks), and symptomatic pseudocysts are indications for drainage, which is best achieved endoscopically or surgically (Ammori & Baghdadi, 2006).

Endoscopic transmural (transgastric or transduodenal) drainage may be possible in some patients with pancreatic pseudocysts, and is best reserved for pseudocysts that complicate chronic pancreatitis (rather than acute pancreatitis) in the head or body of the pancreas, and those with a wall thickness of less than 1cm (Beckingham et al., 1999). Surgery remains the gold standard for the management of large, persistent and recurrent pseudocysts. Internal drainage is conventionally achieved through a pseudocyst-gastrostomy or pseudocyst-jejunostomy, procedures that are now safely and effectively accomplished laparoscopically (Weber et al., 2009). Transgastric (via anterior gastrostomy) (Smadja et al., 1999), endogastric (Mori et al., 2000; Ammori et al., 2002), a posterior approach through the lesser sac, and Roux-en-Y pseudocyst-jejunostomy have been described (Hagopian et al., 2000). Although reported cases of laparoscopic management of pseudocysts are limited, the data presented are promising, and support the advantages of a relatively short postoperative hospital stay and rapid recovery (Smadja et al., 1999; Mori et al., 2000; Ammori et al., 2002; Hagopian et al., 2000).

Because no randomized controlled trial has compared the laparoscopic, open approaches and endoscopic procedures in terms of the internal drainage of pseudocysts, it is impossible to clarify which provides the most effective treatment for patients with pseudocysts in different situations.

5. Conclusion

The anatomical complexity of the pancreas and high postoperative morbidity have hindered evaluations of laparoscopic surgery with respect to early functional recovery, and thus, have probably retarded the adoption of laparoscopic surgery for the management of pancreatic diseases. Nevertheless, recent reports on pancreatic laparoscopic surgery are encouraging and maintain consensus option concerning the merits of the technique.

Well selected cases of enucleation and laparoscopic distal pancreatectomy with or without spleen preservation are currently both acceptable and recommendable for the treatment of benign or low grade malignant diseases of pancreas. Most reports on advanced laparoscopic pancreatectomy have concluded that these procedures are feasible and safe when conducted by skilled laparoscopic surgeons. However, technical feasibility does not obviate sound clinical judgment, and caution should be exercised before new technologies are adopted in the absence of well designed clinical trials (Werner et al., 2005).

Nevertheless many surgeons and the laparoscopic industries have developed new techniques and devices that are more convenient and increase the safety of laparoscopic surgery, and their efforts will undoubtedly increase the role of laparoscopic or minimal invasive surgery for the treatment of pancreatic disease.

6. References

Ammori BJ, Baghdadi S. (2006). Minimally invasive pancreatic surgery: the new frontier? Curr Gastroenterol Rep, Vol.8, No.2, pp. 132-42.

Ammori BJ, Bhattacharya D, Senapati PS. (2002). Laparoscopic endogastric pseudocyst gastrostomy: a report of three cases. Surg Laparosc Endosc Percutan Tech, Vol.12, No.6, pp. 437-40.

Beckingham IJ, Krige JE, Bornman PC, Terblanche J. (1999). Long term outcome of endoscopic drainage of pancreatic pseudocysts. Am J Gastroenterol, Vol.94, No.1, pp. 71-4.

Bergamaschi R, Marvik R, Thoresen JE, Ystgaard B, Johnsen G, Myrvold HE. (1998). Open versus laparoscopic gastrojejunostomy for palliation in advanced pancreatic cancer. Surg Laparosc Endosc, Vol.8, No.2, pp. 92-6.

Brooks AD, Mallis MJ, Brennan MF, Conlon KC. (2002). The value of laparoscopy in the management of ampullary, duodenal, and distal bile duct tumors. J Gastrointest Surg, Vol.6, No.2, pp. 139–145.

Chang YC, Tsai HM, Lin XZ, Chang CH, Chuang JP. (2006). No debridement is necessary for symptomatic or infected acute necrotizing pancreatitis: delayed, mini-retroperitoneal drainage for acute necrotizing pancreatitis without debridement and irrigation. Dig Dis Sci, Vol.51, No.8, pp. 1388-95.

Cho A, Yamamoto H, Nagata M, et al. (2009). Comparison of laparoscopy-assisted and open pylorus-preserving pancreaticoduodenectomy for periampullary disease. Am J Surg, Vol.198, No.3, pp. 445–9.

Cuschieri A. (1996). Laparoscopic pancreatic resections. Semin Laparosc Surg, Vol.3, No.1, pp. 15–20.

DiNorcia J, Schrope BA, Lee MK, et al. (2010). Laparoscopic distal pancreatectomy offers shorter hospital stays with fewer complications. J Gastrointest Surg, Vol.14, No.11, pp. 1804-12.

Doran HE, Bosonnet L, Connor S, et al. (2004). Laparoscopy and laparoscopic ultrasound in the evaluation of pancreatic and periampullary tumours. Dig Surg, Vol.21, No.4, pp. 305–13.

Dulucq JL, Wintringer P, Mahajna A. (2006). Laparoscopic pancreaticoduodenectomy for benign and malignant diseases. Surg Endosc, Vol.20, No.7, pp. 1045–50.

Dulucq JL, Wintringer P, Stabilini C, Feryn T, Perissat J, Mahajna A. (2005). Are major laparoscopic pancreatic resections worthwhile? A prospective study of 32 patients in a single institution. Surg Endosc, Vol.19, No.8, pp. 1028-34.

Eom BW, Jang JY, Lee SE, et al. (2008). Clinical outcomes compared between laparoscopic and open distal pancreatectomy. Surg Endosc, Vol.22, No.5, pp. 1334-8.

Fernandez-Cruz L, Cesar-Borges G, Lopez-Boado MA, Orduna D, Navarro S. (2005). Minimally invasive surgery of the pancreas in progress. Langenbecks Arch Surg, Vol.390, No.4, pp. 342–54.

Fernandez-Cruz L, Cosa R, Blanco L, et al. (2007). Curative laparoscopic resection for pancreatic neoplasms: a critical analysis from a single institution. J Gastrointest Surg, Vol.11, No.12, pp. 1607–21.

Gagner M, Gentileschi P. (2001). Hand-assisted laparoscopic pancreatic resection. Semin Laparosc Surg, Vol.8, No.2, pp. 114-25.

Gagner M, Pomp A. (1994). Laparoscopic pylorus-preserving pancreatoduodenectomy. Surg Endosc, Vol.8, No.5, pp. 408–10.

Gagner M, Pomp A. (1997). Laparoscopic pancreatic resection: is it worthwhile? J Gastrointest Surg, Vol.1, No.1, pp. 20 6.

Garden OJ. (2005). A companion to specialist surgical practice; Hepatobiliary and pancreatic surgery. 3rd ed. Elsevier;.

Giulianotti PC, Sbrana F, Bianco FM, Addeo P, Caravaglios G. (2010). Robot-assisted laparoscopic middle pancreatectomy. J Laparoendosc Adv Surg Tech A, Vol.20, No.2, pp. 135-9.

Hagopian EJ, Texeira JA, Smith M, Steichen FM. (2000). Pancreatic pseudocyst treated by laparoscopic Roux- en-Y cystojejunostomy. Report of a case and review of the literature. Surg Endosc, Vol.14, No.10, p. 967.

Horiguchi A, Uyama I, Ito M, et al. (2011). Robot-assisted laparoscopic pancreatic surgery. J Hepatobiliary Pancreat Sci, Vol.18, No.4, pp. 488-92.

Iihara M, Kanbe M, Okamoto T, Ito Y, Obara T. (2001). Laparoscopic ultrasonography for resection of insulinomas. Surgery, Vol.130, No.6, pp. 1086-91.

Jang JY, Han HS, Yoon YS, Kim SW. (2007). Present status of laparoscopic pancreatic surgery. JIMSA, Vol.20, No.3, pp. 221-25.

Jayaraman S, Gonen M, Brennan MF, D'Angelica MI, DeMatteo RP, Fong Y, JarnaginWR, Allen PJ. (2010). Laparoscopic distal pancreatectomy: evolution of a technique at a single institution. J Am Coll Surg, Vol.211, No.4, pp. 503-9.

Jimenez RE, Warshaw AL, Rattner DW et al. (2000). Impact of laparoscopic staging in the treatment of pancreatic cancer. Arch Surg, Vol.135, No.4, pp. 409–14.

John TG, Wright A, Allan PL et al. (1999). Laparoscopy with laparoscopic ultrasonography in the TNM staging of pancreatic carcinoma. World J Surg, Vol.23, No.9, pp. 870–81.

Kaneko H, Takagi S, Joubara N, et al. (2004). Laparoscopy-assisted spleen-preserving distal pancreatectomy with conservation of the splenic artery and vein. J Hepatobiliary Pancreat Surg, Vol.11, No.6, pp. 397-401.

Kang CM, Kim DH, Lee WJ, Chi HS. (2011). Initial experiences using robot-assisted central pancreatectomy with pancreaticogastrostomy: a potential way to advanced laparoscopic pancreatectomy. Surg Endosc, Vol.25, No.4, pp. 1101-6.

Kendrick ML, Cusati D. (2010). Total laparoscopic pancreaticoduodenectomy: feasibility and outcome in an early experience. Arch Surg, Vol.145, No.1, pp. 19-23.

Kim SC, Park KT, Hwang JW, et al. (2008). Comparative analysis of clinical outcomes for laparoscopic distal pancreatic resection and open distal pancreatic resection at a single institution. Surg Endosc, Vol.22, No.10, pp. 2261–8.

Kooby D, Gillespie T, Bentrem DJ, et al. (2008). Left-sided pancreatectomy: a multicenter comparison of laparoscopic and open approaches. Ann Surg, Vol.248, No.3, pp. 438–46.

Kooby DA, Chu CK. (2010). Laparoscopic management of pancreatic malignancies. Surg Clin North Am, Vol.90, No.2, pp. 427-46.

Kooby DA, Hawkins WG, Schmidt CM, et al. (2010). A multicenter analysis of distal pancreatectomy for adenocarcinoma: is laparoscopic resection appropriate? J Am Coll Surg, Vol.210, No.5, pp. 779-87.

Kubota K. (2011). Recent advances and limitations of surgical treatment for pancreatic cancer. World J Clin Oncol, Vol.2, No.5, pp. 225-8.

Liu RC, Traverso LW. (2005). Diagnostic laparoscopy improves staging of pancreatic cancer deemed locally unresectable by computed tomography. Surg Endosc, Vol.19, No.5, pp. 638–42.

Mabrut JY, Fernandez-Cruz L, Azagra JS, et al. (2005). Laparoscopic pancreatic resection: results of a multicenter European study of 127 patients. Surgery, Vol.137, No.6, pp. 597–605.

Makary MA. (2011). The advent of laparoscopic pancreatic surgery using the robot. Arch Surg, Vol.146, No.3, pp. 261-2.

Mallet GP, Vachon A. (1943). Pancreatites chroniqes gauches. Paris: Masson,.

Matsumoto T, Kitano S, Yoshida T, et al. (1999). Laparoscopic resection of a pancreatic mucinous cystadenoma using laparoscopic coagulating shears. Surg Endosc, Vol.13, No.2, pp. 172–3.

Matsumoto T, Shibata K, Ohta M, et al. (2008). Laparoscopic distal pancreatectomy and open distal pancreatectomy: a nonrandomized comparative study. Surg Laparosc Endosc Percutan Tech, Vol.18, No.4, pp. 340–3.

Melotti G, Butturini G, Piccoli M, et al. (2007). Laparoscopic distal pancreatectomy: results on a consecutive series of 58 patients. Ann Surg, Vol.246, No.1, pp. 77–82.

Menack MJ, Spitz JD, Arregui ME. (2001). Staging of pancreatic and ampullary cancers for resectability using laparoscopy with laparoscopic ultrasound. Surg Endosc, Vol.15, No.10, pp. 1129–34.

Merchant NB, Conlon KC, Saigo P et al. (1999). Positive peritoneal cytology predicts unresectability of pancreatic adenocarcinoma. J Am Coll Surg, Vol.188, No.4, pp. 421–6.

Michl P, Pauls S, Gress TM. (2006). Evidence-based diagnosis and staging of pancreatic cancer. Best Pract Res Clin Gastroenterol, Vol.20, No.2, pp. 227-51.

Minnard EA, Conlon KC, Hoos A et al. (1998). Laparoscopic ultrasound enhances standard laparoscopy in the staging of pancreatic cancer. Ann Surg, Vol.228, No.2, pp. 182–7.

Misawa T, Shiba H, Usuba T, et al. (2007). Systemic inflammatory response syndrome after hand-assisted laparoscopic distal pancreatectomy. Surg Endosc, Vol.21, No.8, pp. 1446–9.

Mori T, Abe N, Sugiyama M, Atomi Y, Way LW. (2000). Laparoscopic pancreatic cystogastrostomy. J Hepatobiliary Pancreat Surg, Vol.7, No.1, pp.28-34.

Mori T, Abe N, Sugiyama M, Atomi Y. (2005). Laparoscopic pancreatic surgery. J Hepatobiliary Pancreat Surg, Vol.12, No.6, pp. 451-5.

Nakamura Y, Uchida E, Aimoto T, et al. (2009). Clinical outcome of laparoscopic distal pancreatectomy. J Hepatobiliary Pancreat Surg, Vol.16, No.1, pp. 35–41.

Nieveen van Dijkum EJ, de Wit LT, van Delden OM et al. (1999). Staging laparoscopy and laparoscopic ultrasonography in more than 400 patients with upper gastrointestinal carcinoma. J Am Coll Surg, Vol.189, No.5, pp. 459–65.

Nieveen van Dijkum EJ, Romijn MG, Terwee CB et al. (2003). Laparoscopic staging and subsequent palliation in patients with peripancreatic carcinoma. Ann Surg, Vol.237, No.1, pp. 66–73.

Orsenigo E, Baccari P, Bissolotti G, Staudacher C. (2006). Laparoscopic central pancreatectomy. Am J Surg, Vol.191, No.4, pp. 549-52.

Palanivelu C, Shetty R, Jani K, et al. (2007). Laparoscopic distal pancreatectomy: results of a prospective non-randomized study from a tertiary center. Surg Endosc, Vol.21, No.3, pp. 373–7.

Parekh D. (2006). Laparoscopic-assisted pancreatic necrosectomy: A new surgical option for treatment of severe necrotizing pancreatitis. Arch Surg, Vol.141, No.9, pp. 895-902.

Pugliese R, Scandroglio I, Sansonna F, et al. (2008). Laparoscopic pancreaticoduodenectomy: a retrospective review of 19 cases. Surg Laparosc Endosc Percutan Tech, Vol.18, No.1, pp. 13–8.

Pyke CM, van Heerden JA, Colby TV, Sarr MG, Weaver AL. (1992). The spectrum of serous cystadenoma of the pancreas. Clinical, pathologic, and surgical aspects. Ann Surg, Vol.215, No.2, pp. 132–9.

Rhodes M, Nathanson L, Fielding G. (1995). Laparoscopic biliary and gastric bypass: a useful adjunct in the treatment of carcinoma of the pancreas. Gut, Vol.36, No.5, pp. 778-80.

Robey E, Mullen JT, Schwab CW. (1982). Blunt trisection of the pancreas treated by distal pancreatectomy, splenic salvage and hyperalimentation. Four cases and review of the literature. Ann Surg, Vol.196, No.6, pp. 695-9.

Røsok BI, Marangos IP, Kazaryan AM, et al. (2010). Single-centre experience of laparoscopic pancreatic surgery. Br J Surg, Vol.97, No.6 , pp. 902-9.

Rothlin MA, Schob O, Weber M. (1999). Laparoscopic gastro- and hepaticojejunostomy for palliation of pancreatic cancer: a case controlled study. Surg Endosc, Vol.13, No.11, pp. 1065-9.

Schachter PP, Avni Y, Shimonov M, et al. (2000). The impact of laparoscopy and laparoscopic ultrasonography on the management of pancreatic cancer. Arch Surg, Vol.135, No.11, pp. 1303-7.

Schwarz A, Beger HG. (2000). Biliary and gastric bypass or stenting in nonresectable periampullary cancer: analysis on the basis of controlled trials. Int J Pancreatol, Vol.27, No.1, pp. 51-8.

Smadja C, Badawy A, Vons C, Giraud V, Franco D. (1999). Laparoscopic cystogastrostomy for pancreatic pseudocyst is safe and effective. J Laparoendosc Adv Surg Tech A, Vol.9, No.5, pp. 401-3.

Song KB, Kim SC, et al. (2011). Single-center experience of laparoscopic left pancreatic resection in 359 consecutive patients: changing the surgical paradigm of left pancreatic resection. Surg Endosc, May 10.

Staudacher C, Orsenigo E, Baccari P, et al. (2005). Laparoscopic assisted duodenopancreatectomy. Surg Endosc, Vol.19, No.3, pp. 352–6.

Tagaya N, Kasama K, Suzuki N, Taketsuka S, Horie K, Furihata M, Kubota K. (2003). Laparoscopic resection of the pancreas and review of the literature. Surg Endosc, Vol.17, No.2, pp. 201-6.

Talamini MA, Moesinger R, Yeo CJ, Poulose B, Hruban RH, Cameron JL, Pitt HA. (1998). Cystadenomas of the pancreas: is enucleation an adequate operation? Ann Surg, Vol.227, No.6, pp. 896–903.

Teh SH, Tseng D, Sheppard BC. (2007). Laparoscopic and open distal pancreatic resection for benign pancreatic disease. J Gastrointest Surg, Vol.11, No.9, pp. 1120–5.

van den Bosch RP, van der Schelling GP, Klinkenbijl JH, Mulder PG, van Blankenstein M, Jeekel J. (1994). Guidelines for the application of surgery and endoprostheses in the palliation of obstructive jaundice in advanced cancer of the pancreas. Ann Surg, Vol.219, No.1, pp. 18-24.

Velanovich V. (2006). Case-control comparison of laparoscopic versus open distal pancreatectomy. J Gastrointest Surg, Vol.10, No.1, pp. 95–8.

Velasco JM, Rossi H, Hieken TJ, Fernandez M. (2000). Laparoscopic ultrasound enhances diagnostic laparoscopy in the staging of intra-abdominal neoplasms. Am Surg, Vol.66, No.4, pp. 407–11.

Vijan SS, Ahmed KA, Harmsen WS, et al. (2010). Laparoscopic vs open distal pancreatectomy: a single-institution comparative study. Arch Surg, Vol.145, No.7, pp. 616-21.

Warshaw A. (1997). Techniques of preserving the spleen with distal pancreatectomy. Surgery, Vol.121, p. 974.

Weber SM, Cho CS, Merchant N, et al. (2009). Laparoscopic left pancreatectomy:complication risk score correlates with morbidity and risk for pancreatic fistula. Ann Surg Oncol, Vol.16, No.10, pp. 2825-33.

Werner J, Feuerbach S, Uhi W, Buchler MW. (2005.)Management of acute pancreatitis: from surgery to interventional intensive care. Gut, Vol.54, No.3, pp. 426-36.

Yamaguchi K, Noshiro H, Yokohata K, et al. (2001). Is there any benefit of preservation of the spleen in distal pancreatectomy? Int Surg, Vol.86, No.3, pp. 162-8.

Yoon YS, Lee KH, Han HS, Cho JY, Ahn KS. (2009). Patency of splenic vessels after laparoscopic spleen and splenic vessel-preserving distal pancreatectomy. Br J Surg, Vol.96, No.6, pp. 633-40.

4

Laparoscopy in Trauma Patients

Cino Bendinelli[1] and Zsolt J. Balogh[1,2]
[1]*John Hunter Hospital, Newcastle, NSW,*
[2]*University of Newcastle, NSW,*
Australia

1. Introduction

The burden of major trauma, predominantly blunt in nature, continues to rise in most countries. More often the young are affected with lifelong debilitating consequences. Minimally invasive techniques, such as laparoscopic procedures, have become standard for the treatment of many surgical conditions, being able to minimize the impact of surgery, to reduce postoperative pain, time in hospital, time to recover, and to improve cosmetic outcomes.

The use of laparoscopy as an aid in the diagnosis of abdominal trauma was first described in 1977 (Simon, Gazzaniga, Carnevale). In 1988 Cuschieri compared diagnostic peritoneal lavage with a laparoscopy (using a 4-mm scope) in blunt abdominal trauma patients demonstrating that laparoscopy carried a higher positive predictive value when compared to diagnostic peritoneal lavage (Cuschieri). Since then, the use of laparoscopy in abdominal trauma has increased exponentially. In trauma patients laparoscopy may avoid unnecessary (non-therapeutic) laparotomy, may improve operative visualisation of diaphragm, and may allow laparoscopic repair of these injuries.

Despite these clear potentialities, laparoscopy has not yet gained wide acceptation and it is not consistently performed in trauma patients. There are several reasons for this.

1. In bleeding, or potentially bleeding patients, timing is of essence. The logistics for laparoscopy set up of theatre still takes longer than for open surgery. Once the operation has started it takes longer to gain access, identify the bleeder and, especially, control it when compared to a trauma laparotomy.
2. In haemodynamically normal patients with spleen injuries a diagnostic laparoscopy may increase the splenectomy rate.
3. The risk of missing injuries (hollow viscus mainly) is high. A literature review reports a 41% to 77% rate of missed injuries when used as a diagnostic tool to perform abdominal exploration (Villavicencio). This is very much operator dependent, but it may carry disastrous outcomes.
4. Logistics wise most trauma happens at night when staff may be less motivated to embark in a time consuming procedure.

2. Indication

In trauma patients laparoscopy maybe used either as a diagnostic or as a therapeutic tool. Both are generally indicated only for patients with normal hemodynamics and in which major bleeding is not expected.

3. Diagnostic laparoscopy

Exploratory laparotomy in either blunt or penetrating abdominal trauma patients with suspected intra-abdominal injuries is associated with a high negative (non-therapeutic) laparotomy rate and a high procedure-related morbidity (41% according to Renz). Diagnostic laparoscopy in trauma patients is reported to spare a median of 57% (range, 17–89%) of non-therapeutic laparotomy (Stefanidis). Depending on centres, indications for diagnostic laparoscopy varies widely including suspected intraabdominal injury after blunt trauma, abdominal stab wounds with proven or equivocal penetration of fascia, abdominal gunshot wounds with doubtful intraperitoneal trajectory, diagnosis of diaphragmatic injury from penetrating trauma to the thoracoabdominal area, and creation of a transdiaphragmatic pericardial window to rule out cardiac injury. The sensitivity, specificity, and diagnostic accuracy of diagnostic laparoscopy when used to predict the need for laparotomy range from 75 to 100% (Hori). When diagnostic laparoscopy has been used as a screening tool (conversion to laparotomy with the first encounter of a positive finding: peritoneal penetration in penetrating trauma or free blood in blunt trauma patients), the number of missed injuries is <1% (Hori). For penetrating trauma a sensitivity of 80–100%, specificity of 38–86%, and accuracy of 54–89% have been consistently reported (Villavicnezio, Leppaniemi).

Most trauma centres include diagnostic laparoscopy in the algorithm for management of patients with penetrating thoraco-abdominal trauma (Fig 1) (Biffl, Sugrue, Zantut, Lin, Mallat, Fabian). Patients without signs of shock, evisceration, or peritonitis undergo a "screening laparoscopy" to identify peritoneal or diaphragmatic penetration. In this setting screening laparoscopy is a better tool compared to local wound exploration (especially in large body habitus, uncooperative patient and thoraco abdominal injuries). Diaphragmatic injuries occur in up to 20% of patients with penetrating thoracoabdominal trauma (Friese, Powel). These are often undetected, remain clinically silent, only to present later with life-threatening complications associated with diaphragmatic herniation. Diagnostic laparoscopy is not useful in posterior abdominal wall penetration to rule out retroperitoneal injuries.

An extension of diagnostic laparoscopy includes laparoscopic pericardial window for exclusion of cardiac injury in patients with thoracoabdominal penetrating wounds, normal hemodynamic status and free pericardial fluid at ultrasound. The pericardial membrane needs to be incised with endoshears and electrocautery must not be used to prevent possible dysrhythmia or myocardial damage (McMahon).

Following blunt abdominal trauma hemodynamic instability and a positive FAST (Focused Abdominal Sonography in Trauma) or Diagnostic Peritoneal Aspiration mandates immediate midline laparotomy. Laparoscopy may play a role in patients with blunt abdominal trauma, who are not bleeding, but have unclear findings on CT (bowel wall thickening, stranding of the mesentery, dilated bowel loops, extraluminal retroperitoneal air and/or free fluid without solid organ injury) and the patient's clinical status is only suspicious or not assessable (comatose patients). In this subgroup of patients delay in diagnosis occurs in up to 5% of cases and contributes to increased morbidity from 10 to 30% (Mathonet). Laparoscopy for blunt trauma reported a sensitivity of 90–100%, specificity of 86–100%, and accuracy of 88–100% for bowel injuries (Villavicencio and Aucar)

Findings of FAST can be categorised into three groups: those without injuries, those with injuries who do not require surgical treatment, and those who require repair which may be accomplished laparoscopically depending on the laparoscopic skills of the surgeon.

4. Therapeutic laparoscopy

The guidelines for diagnostic laparoscopy, published by the Society of American Gastrointestinal and Endoscopic Surgeons, stated that diagnostic laparoscopy is contraindicated when there is obvious intra-abdominal injury or peritonitis (Hori).

Many AA have challenged this and, over the last 20 years, sporadic groups, with a specific interest in laparoscopy, have first demonstrated FAST to be a safe and consistent diagnostic tool in both blunt and penetrating trauma and then proved therapeutic laparoscopy to be safe in repairing the encountered injuries.

Laparoscopic repairs of injuries to virtually every organ have been described. Injuries to diaphragm (Simon), parenchymal organs and gastro-intestinal tract (Cherkasov, Lin) have been successfully repaired laparoscopically. Large case series exist from institutions that provide full definitive laparoscopic management of any injuries (also in shocked and actively bleeding patients) with no or minimal missed injuries and dismal conversion rate (Cherkasov, Lin).

Actively bleeding spleen injuries may be treated laparoscopically. Patients who continue to bleed following embolization or with high grade spleen injuries are treated with laparoscopic application of collagen-fibrinogen human thrombin seal on oozing lacerations and if a major bleeding is encountered laparoscopic splenectomy is then performed (Olmi, Marzano).

Non-operative management of hepatic and splenic injuries is successful in up to 80% of instances. Many of these patients (up to 75% in high grade injuries) will demonstrate signs of inflammatory response due to the haemoperitoneum (fever, leukocytosis, discomfort, and tachycardia) (Letoublon). The use of laparoscopy to remove the old blood from the peritoneal cavity maybe accomplished safely and maybe beneficial (Carillo). During the procedure the solid organs and the clots on their surface are left alone to avoid any potential haemorrhage. Bilioma and biliary peritonitis due to bile duct injuries may also be treated with collagen-fibrinogen human thrombin seal and/or drained laparoscopically. (Carillo Sugrue, Marzano).

Small lacerations of stomach, duodenum, small bowel, and colon can be repaired laparoscopically. When an anastomosis or a long repair is required these are usually performed extracorporeally through a small focused celiotomy (Hope Streck, Ianelli).

5. Contraindication

Although some centres have questioned it (Cherkasov) haemodynamic instability is currently the absolute contraindication for laparoscopy. The main reason for this is that bleeding identification and control cannot be performed rapidly by laparoscopic means (Ball, Hori).

Concomitant severe traumatic brain injury should also exclude laparoscopy. Some animal models (Goetler), case reports (Mobbs), and extrapolation from series of patients with abdominal compartment syndrome suggest that intracerebral pressure maybe increased by high abdominal pressures (Joseph).

Contraindications such as previous abdominal scars are relative, as optical port can create a safe access, but if intraabdominal adhesions prevent full and confident exploration the procedure should be converted.

Tension pneumothorax is always a possible complication when a diaphragmatic injury allows CO2 to fill the pleural cavity. As discussed above, this is diagnosed earlier when using low flow rate for induction of pneumoperitoneum and best treated with prompt chest drain insertion. A chest drain should always be available during the procedure (Ball).

One of the most important contraindication will always be lack of inadequate laparoscopic skills. A screening laparoscopy to rule out peritoneal violation is an easy task, full abdominal exploration is a time consuming challenging procedure, and laparoscopic repair of bowel an advanced laparoscopic skill.

6. Technique

Positioning and preparation of the patient for trauma laparoscopy is essentially the same as for any trauma laparotomy. The theatre is warm and instruments for a conversion to laparotomy or access to the thorax should readily available. The patient is placed supine on a beanbag and well strapped. Bed tilting is crucial to allow gravity to retract abdominal organs and to increase working space. Pneumoperitoneum is achieved with low CO2 flow and maintained at low pressures (8-12 mmHg). Low flow rate allows timely detection of a tension pneumothorax (increased ventilatory pressures and/or hypotension). Should this occur the pneumoperitoneum is immediately released and a size 32Fr chest drain is inserted on the most likely side. The procedure is then carried out open (Fabian).

Diagnositc laparoscopy is achieved trough a 10mm umbilical port best inserted with an open technique. A 30degree laparoscope (5-10mm in diameter) allows optimal visualization of abdominal wall, diaphrams and liver/spleen dome. Tilting the bed in Trendelenburg position or reverse Trendelenburg position allows visualization of lower and upper abdomen. For paracolic gutters exploration lateral tilting is required. In the case of penetrating wounds, air leaks trough the skin may need to be controlled with sutures or external digital pressure. In most cases visceral handling is necessary and easily carried out with 5mm atraumatic bowel graspers through two paramedian 5mm ports placed on the umbilical line. A 5mm laparoscope (which carries less light and may be inadequate in bloody fields) allows liberal interchange of the instruments between the ports. Peritoneal violation can be determined easily and reliably.

Performing a full laparoscopic exploration of the abdominal cavity in search for injuries requires a systematic approach which follows all principles of open exploratory laparotomy (Kawahara). Indirect signs of bowel injury, such as digestive fluids or purulent liquids must be carefully looked for. Methylene blue administered IV or via the nasogastric tube may help to identify urologic or proximal bowel injuries. Some AA advocate laparoscopic assisted diagnostic peritoneal lavage to rule out bowel injuries trough absence of alkaline phosphatase, bile or fibers in the lavage. This concept may add to diagnostic laparoscopy sensitivity in excluding gut injuries and make most trauma surgeon more confident in adopting it.

The bowel requires to be examined using the hand-over-hand technique with small bowel graspers from the ligament of Treitz to the terminal ileum. The colon is inspected from the cecum to the rectum and the supramesocolic space is inspected from the abdominal esophagus to the duodenum including spleen, liver and gallbladder. A laparoscopic full Kocher manoeuvre is accomplished in right lateral decubitus, the hepatic flexure of the colon is mobilized to the left side using the harmonic scalpel. The peritoneum is incised lateral to duodenum and blunt dissection mobilizes the duodenum medially in order to explore its dorsal aspect (Gorecki, Cherkasov, Kawahara, Lin).

For therapeutic laparoscopy more ports are usually necessary and usually titrated based on the surgical procedure required and the size of the patient. Extensive laparoscopic expertise is mandatory, to be able to treat patients with intestinal perforations. Laparoscopic suturing of bowel injuries is carried out with either silk or Vycril suture (Hope, Tytgal). An extra port may be necessary to achieve lining up of the bowel. If possible the bowel should be inflated and the suture line submerged in saline to rule out air leaks. Diaphragm repairs are best achieved with braided non absorbable sutures and large needles.

For splenectomy 4 ports are necessary: one 10-mm umbilical port, two 5-mm ports at left subcostal margin (for retraction and irrigation purposes); a 12-mm port below the left subcostal margin at mid-clavicular line. Right lateral tilting of the bed and reverse Trendelenberg allow suspending the spleen for optimal laparoscopic visualization. Subcapsular hematomas and coagulum are not disturbed to minimize bleeding. Using the harmonic scalpel (or Ligasure) the splenocolic ligament is first taken down from the lower pole of the spleen. The gastrosplenic ligament with short gastrics is then divided with harmonic scalpel (or Ligasure). The splenic hilum is secured and divided with several applications of a 35-mm linear endovascular stapling device. Prompt conversion may be necessary if massive bleeding is encountered. Hand assistance, with a hand port in order to control the hilar blood vessels (Ren) may be handy! This is particularly true when active bleeding is obscuring the field or when the endovascular stapling device fails.

Hand assistance can be performed readily and should be considered a potential adjunct to minimally invasive surgical procedure.

Conversion to celiotomy is mandated when visceral exploration is not adequate (obesity or tenacious postoperative adherences), or when hemodynamic instability arises during laparoscopy. Although laparoscopy does offer potential benefits, the trauma surgeon should never let the lure of a "minimally invasive" procedure compromise patient care or the use of sound clinical judgment.

7. Sequale of trauma

Laparoscopy is a well validated technique to repair abdominal wall and diaphragmatic defects, which may follow blunt or penetrating trauma. These procedures are less controversial and considered safer mainly because they are carried out as elective procedures, with a clear plan in terms of ports placement and methods of repair. There is usually no need to explore the abdomen in search for other injuries. Diaphragmatic defects are best repaired with direct suture. When the defect is too large an expanded polytetrafluoroethylene or double layered prosthesis is utilized (Matz, Baldassarre). The mesh is secured with a combination of endoscopic tacks and laparoscopic suturing (Bobbio). Endoscopic tacks should not be used on the diaphragm, due to the risks of lung and heart injury (Bendinelli).

8. Future

The future holds exciting advances for this field of surgery through innovative developments. All AA agree that an improvement in instrumentation is still required. In the near future laparoscopic management of abdominal trauma will play a greater role in the treatment of haemodynamically stable patients and might one day be a reasonable option for unstable patients.

Further research needs to analyse outcome measures of laparoscopic techniques in comparison to traditional laparotomy. The beneficial effect of laparoscopic treatment of injuries should be investigated further before the widespread adoption of this approach.

The main concern will always be missed injuries. To minimize the risk of missing bowel injuries it might be worth to combine explorative laparoscopy with laparoscopic lavage using the standard laboratory criteria (Otomo). This concept, which is definitely intriguing although logistically demanding, warrants further evaluation (Vinces).

The learning curve typical of any procedure (especially laparoscopic ones) will have to be better understood. Adequate training and support to Trauma Surgeon should be provided by dedicated laparoscopists both in Operating Theatre and in *ad hoc* courses.

With the current obese pandemia laparoscopy may be even more beneficial, as many penetrating injuries do not reach the abdominal cavity or if they do organs may be more protected by thick omentum. This must be compared to the higher morbidity rate of a full midline laparotomy in obese patients.

Screening laparoscopy for penetrating abdominal trauma using only local anaesthetics can be performed in the Emergency Department in awake patients (Weinberg). Laparoscopy may become a triage tool in Emergency Department (discharge versus laparotomy) and would be of great value in busy metropolitan Trauma Centres.

Laparoscopy typically minimizes the insult of surgery and may also play a role in reducing the incidence of Systemic inflammatory response syndrome (SIRS) often seen in multiple injured trauma patients.

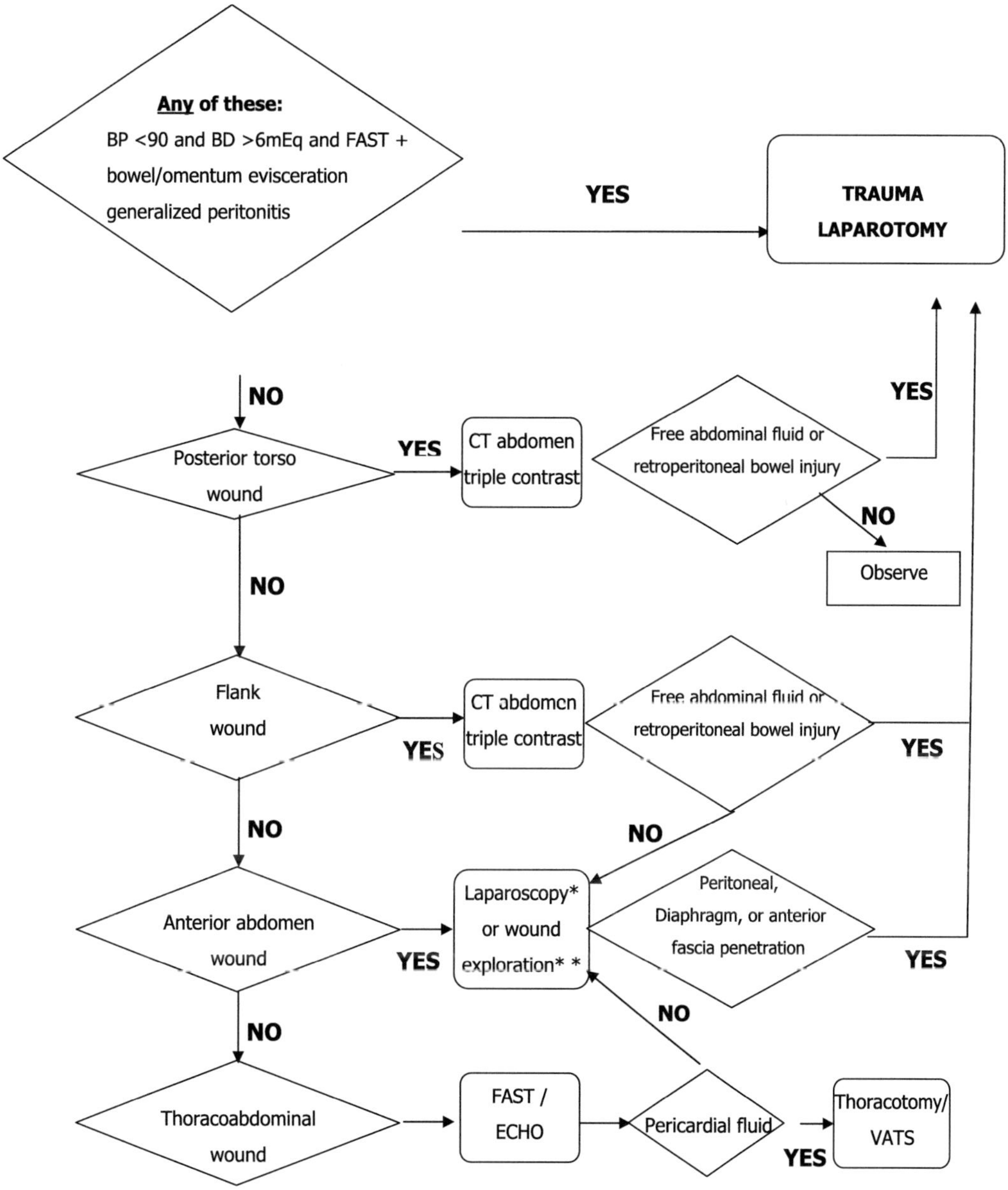

*Wound exploration is recommended only in thin and cooperative patients.

Fig. 1. Institutional guidelines for penetrating torso trauma

9. References

Baldassarre E, Valenti G, Gambino M, Arturi A, Torino G, Porta IP, Barone M. The role of laparoscopy in the diagnosis and the treatment of missed diaphragmatic hernia after penetrating trauma. J Laparoendosc Adv Surg Tech A. 2007;17:302-6.

Ball CG, Kirkpatrick AW. Intra-abdominal hypertension and the abdominal compartment syndrome. Scand J Surg 2007;96:197–204.

Bendinelli C, Martin A, Balogh ZJ. Strangulated intercostal liver herniation subsequent to blunt trauma. First report with review of the world literature. Staged management and laparoscopic repair. ANZjS: 2012 (in press).

Biffl WL, Moore EE. Management guidelines for penetrating abdominal trauma. Curr Opin Crit Care. 2010 Sep (in press)

Bobbio, L. Ampollini, G. Prinzi, et al. Endoscopic Repair of an Abdominal Intercostal Hernia. Surg Laparosc Endosc Percutan Tech 2008; 18:523–525.

Carnevale N, Baron N, Delaney HM. Peritoneoscopy as an aid in the diagnosis of abdominal trauma: a preliminary report. J Trauma 1977; 17:634-41.

Carobbi A, Romagnani F, Antonelli G, Bianchini M. Laparoscopic splenectomy for severe blunt trauma: initial experience of ten consecutive cases with a fast hemostatic technique. Surg Endosc. 2010;24:1325-30.

Carrillo EH, Reed DN Jr, Gordon L, Spain DA, Richardson JD. Delayed laparoscopy facilitates the management of biliary peritonitis in patients with complex liver injuries. Surg Endosc 2001, 15:319-22.

Cherkasov M, Sitnikov V, Sarkisyan B, Degtirev O, Turbin M, Yakuba ALaparoscopy versus laparotomy in management of abdominal trauma. Surg Endosc. 2008;22:228-31

Como JJ, Bokhari F, Chiu WC, Duane TM, Holevar MR, Tandoh MA, Ivatury RR, Scalea TM. Practice management guidelines for selective nonoperative management of penetrating abdominal trauma. J Trauma. 2010;68:721-33.

Cui H, Luckeroth P, Peralta R. Laparoscopic management of penetrating liver trauma: a safe intervention for hemostasis. J Laparoendosc Adv Surg Tech A. 2007;17:219 –222.

Cuschieri A, Hennessy TP, Stephens RB, Berci G. Diagnosis of significant abdominal trauma after road traffic accidents: preliminary results of a multicentre clinical trial comparing minilaparoscopy with peritoneal lavage. Ann R Coll Surg Engl. 1988;70:153-5.

Degiannis E,Bowley DM,Smith MD. Minimally invasive surgery in trauma: technology looking for an application. Injury2004;35:474–8.

Fabian TC, Croce MA, Stewart RM, Pritchard FE, Minard G, Kudsk KA. A prospective analysis of diagnostic laparoscopy in trauma. Ann Surg. 1993;217:557-65.

Feliz A, Shultz B, McKenna C,Gaines BA. Diagnostic and therapeutic laparoscopy in pediatric abdominal trauma. J Pediatr Surg 2006;41:72–7.

Friese RS, Coln CE, Gentilello LM. Laparoscopy is sufficient to exclude occult diaphragm injury after penetrating abdominal trauma. J Trauma. 2005;58:789-92.

Gaines BA, Rutkoski JD. The role of laparoscopy in pediatric trauma. Semin Pediatr Surg. 2010;19:300-3.

Gazzaniga AB, Slanton WEW, Bartlett RH. Laparoscopy in the diagnosis of blunt and penetrating injuries to the abdomen. Am J Surg 1976; 131:315-18.

Goettler CE, Bard MR, Toschlog EA. Laparoscopy in trauma. Curr Surg 2004;61:554–9.

Gorecki PJ, Cottam D, Angus LDG, et al. Diagnostic and therapeutic laparoscopyfor trauma: a technique of safe and systematic exploration. Surg Laparosc Endosc Percutan Tech 2002;12:195–8.

Hope WW, Christmas AB,Dg Jacobs, RF Sing. Definitive laparoscopic repair of penetrating injuries to the colon and small intestine: A Case Report. J Trauma. 2009;66:931–932.

Hori Y; SAGES Guidelines Committee. Diagnostic laparoscopy guidelines : This guideline was prepared by the SAGES Guidelines Committee and reviewed and approved by the Board of Governors of the Society of American Gastrointestinal and Endoscopic Surgeons (SAGES), November 2007. Surg Endosc. 2008;22:1353-83.

Huscher CGS, Mingoli A, Sgarzini G, Brachini G, Ponzano C, Di Paola M, Mondini C Laparoscopic treatment of blunt splenic injuries: initial experience with 11 patients. Surg Endosc 2006;20:1423–1426.

Iannelli A, Fabiani P, Karimdjee BS, Baque P, Venissac N, Gugenheim J. Therapeutic laparoscopy for blunt abdominal trauma with bowel injuries. J Laparoendosc Adv Surg Tech A. 2003;13:189–191.

Joseph DK, Dutton RP, Aarabi B, Scalea TM. Decompressive laparotomy to treat intractable intracranial hypertension after traumatic brain injury. J Trauma. 2004; 57:687-95.

Kawahara NT, Alster C, Fujimura I, Poggetti RS, Birolini D. Standard examination system for laparoscopy in penetrating abdominal trauma. J Trauma. 2009;67:3:589-95.

Leppaniemi A, Haapiainen R Diagnostic laparoscopy in abdominal stab wounds: a prospective, randomized study. J Trauma 2003; 54):636-45.

Letoublon C, Chen Y, Arvieux C, Voirin D, Morra I, Broux C, Risse O. Delayed celiotomy or laparoscopy as part of the nonoperative management of blunt hepatic trauma. World J Surg. 2008;32:1189-93.

Lin HF, Wu JM, Tu CC, Chen HA, Shih HC. Value of diagnostic and therapeutic laparoscopy for abdominal stab wounds. World J Surg. 2010;34:1653-62.

Livingston DH, Lavery RF, Passannante MR, Skurnick JH, Baker S, Fabian TC, Fry DE, Malangoni MA. Free fluid on abdominal computed tomography without solid organ injury after blunt abdominal injury does not mandate celiotomy. Am J Surg 2001; 182: 6–9.

Mallat AF, Mancini ML, Daley BJ, Enderson BL. The role of laparoscopy in trauma: a ten-year review of diagnosis and therapeutics. Am Surg. 2008;74:1166-70.

Marks JM, Youngelman DF, Berk T. Cost analysis of diagnostic laparoscopy vs laparotomy in the evaluation of penetrating abdominal trauma. Surg Endosc. 1997;11:272-6.

Marzano E, Rosso E, Oussoultzoglou E, Collange O, Bachellier P, Pessaux P. Laparoscopic treatment of biliary peritonitis following nonoperative management of blunt liver trauma. World Journal of Emergency Surgery 2010, 5:26.

Matz A, Landau O, Alis M, Charuzi I, Kyzer S. The role of laparoscopy in the diagnosis and treatment of missed diaphragmatic rupture. Surg Endosc. 2000;14:537-9.

McMahon DJ, Sing RF, Hoff WS, Schwab CW. Laparoscopic transdiaphragmatic diagnostic pericardial window in the hemodynamically stable patient with penetrating chest trauma. A brief report. Surg Endosc. 1997;11:474-5.

Mobbs RJ, Ow Yang M. The dangers of diagnostic laparoscopy in the head injured patient. J Clin Neurosci 2002;9:592–3.

Nasr WI, Collins CL, Kelly JJ. Feasibility of laparoscopic splenectomy in stable blunt trauma: a case series. J Trauma. 2004; 57:887– 889.

Olmi S, Scaini A, Erba L, Bertolini A, Guaglio M, Croce E. Use of fibrin glue (Tissucol) as a hemostatic in laparoscopic conservative treatment of spleen trauma. Surg Endosc. 2007;21:2051-4.

Otomo Y, Henmi H, Mashiko K, Kato K, Koike K, Koido Y, Kimura A, Honma M, Inoue J, Yamamoto Y. New diagnostic peritoneal lavage criteria for diagnosis of intestinal injury. J Trauma 1998;44: 131–139.

Powell BS, Magnotti LJ, Schroeppel TJ, Finnell CW, Savage SA, Fischer PE, Fabian TC, Croce MA. Diagnostic laparoscopy for the evaluation of occult diaphragmatic injury following penetrating thoracoabdominal trauma. Injury. 2008;39:530-4.

Pucci E, Brody F, Zemon H, Ponsky T, Venbrux A. Laparoscopic splenectomy for delayed splenic rupture after embolization. J Trauma 2007;63:687–690.

Renz BM, Feliciano DV. Unnecessary laparotomies for trauma: a prospective study of morbidity. J Trauma 1995;38:350–6.

Simon RJ, Rabin J, Kuhls D. Impact of increased use of laparoscopy on negative laparotomy rates after penetrating trauma. J Trauma. 2002;53:297-302.

Sitnikov V, Yakubu A, Sarkisyan V, Turbin M.The role of video-assisted laparoscopy in management of patients with small bowel injuries in abdominal trauma. Surg Endosc. 2009;23:125-9.

Stefanidis D, Richardson WS, Chang L, Earle DB, Fanelli RD. The role of diagnostic laparoscopy for acute abdominal conditions: an evidence-based review. Surg Endosc. 2009;23:16-23.

Streck CJ, Lobe TE, Pietsch JB, Lovvorn HN III. Laparoscopic repair of traumatic bowel injury in children. J Pediatr Surg. 2006;41:1864–1869.

Sugrue M, Balogh Z, Lynch J, Bardsley J, Sisson G, Weigelt J. Guidelines for the management of haemodynamically stable patients with stab wounds to the anterior abdomen. ANZ J Surg. 2007;77:614-20.

Tytgat SH, Zwaveling S, Kramer WL, van der Zee DC. Laparoscopic treatment of gastric and duodenal perforation in children after blunt abdominal trauma. Injury. 2010 Dec (in press)

Uranüs S, Dorr K. Laparoscopy in Abdominal Trauma. Eur J Trauma Emerg Surg 2010; 1.

Villavicencio RT, Aucar JA. Analysis of laparoscopy in trauma. J Am Coll Surg. 1999;189:11-20.

Vinces FY, Madlinger RV. Laparoscopic exploration and lavage in penetrating abdominal stab wounds: a preliminary report. Ulus Travma Acil Cerrahi Derg. 2009;15:109-12.

Weinberg JA, Magnotti LJ, Edwards NM, Claridge JA, Minard G, Fabian TC, Croce MA. "Awake" laparoscopy for the evaluation of equivocal penetrating abdominal wounds. Injury. 2007;38:60-4.

Zantut LF, Ivatury RR, Smith RS, Kawahara NT, Porter JM, Fry WR, Poggetti R, Birolini D, Organ CH Jr. Diagnostic and therapeutic laparoscopy for penetrating abdominal trauma: a multicenter experience. J Trauma. 1997;42:825-31.

Part 2

Urology Procedures

5

Laparoscopic Ureteroureterostomy

Oner Sanli, Tzevat Tefik and Selcuk Erdem
Department of Urology, Istanbul Faculty of Medicine, Istanbul University, Turkey

1. Introduction

Ureter is the conduit carrying urine from renal pelvis to bladder. Since it has long course; many extrinsic pathologies, intrinsic mural anomalies and luminal defects may affect continuity of the ureter. Ureteric reconstruction aims to achieve integrity of the urinary tract in pathological conditions while preserving renal function. However, ureteric reconstruction is one of the challenging procedures in urology since the length and location of the problematic ureter or underlying pathology does not allow performing one kind of surgery in all situations.

The level of ureteral disease is indicative to make a decision on appropriate reconstructive procedure. The repair of 2/3 proximal ureter located above the pelvic brim is generally more demanding. Ureteroureteral anastomosis (ureteroureterostomy) is a suitable procedure for short pathologies located in the mid- and proximal ureter; meanwhile transureteroureterostomy, ureteral substitution and renal autotransplantation techniques are useful for large affected ureteral disease. (Png & Chapple, 2000) On the other hand, ureteroneocyctostomy, Boari's flap or psoas hitch procedures are well-accepted treatment alternatives for the 1/3 distal part of ureter below the pelvic brim. All techniques may be performed with open, laparoscopic and robot-assisted laparoscopic approaches.

In the last 20 years, urological community witnessed a revolution that; traditional open surgery has been largely replaced by endoscopic and laparoscopic techniques. This radical leap has gained widespread acceptance due to well-documented advantages of minimally invasive surgery. Since the introduction of laparoscopy in the field of urology, the number of centers performing this approach has been increasing steadily. It is acknowledged that laparoscopy provides surgical outcomes with efficacy equal to that of open surgery. (Guillonneau et al., 2001) For this reason, more clinics are adapting the trend of laparoscopy. Due to the clear advantages of laparoscopic surgery, the indications of this approach have expanded dramatically over the years. (Dunn et al., 2000) Similarly, the renowned benefits of minimal invasive surgery such as less pain, quicker convalescence and improved cosmesis are also well perceived by the patients. Moreover, decreased intra-operative blood loss, lesser need of transfusions and shortened hospital stay makes this approach as a *"sine qua non"* of the current and future urologic surgery.

Even though, laparoscopic ureteroureterostomy (LUU) has been performed in major tertiary centers, where the surgeons facile with laparoscopic techniques and perfect surgery; the wide application of laparoscopy in many centers throughout the world encourages experienced surgical teams to perform challenging procedures such as LUU. Accordingly, this chapter will focus on LUU performed for relatively small pathologies that affect proximal 2/3 part of ureter.

2. Laparoscopic anatomy of ureter

The ureter when measured from the ureteropelvic junction (UPJ) to the bladder is about 28 to 34 cm long. Anatomically, the ureter is divided in three segments. The proximal ureter extends from the UPJ to the area where the ureter crosses sacroiliac joint, the middle ureter courses over the bony pelvis and the distal ureter extends from the iliac vessels to the bladder. (Pereira et al., 2010) Each ureter passes over the medial part of the psoas major in the line with the ends of the transverse processes of the lumbar vertebrae. Then they cross the genitofemoral nerve and pass under the gonadal vessels into the pelvis near the bifurcation of the common iliac vessels (CIVs). After crossing the CIVs, the ureters follow the course of internal iliac artery and run along the anterior border of the greater sciatic notch. Thereupon, they turn medially at the ischial spine and lie along the levator ani just before entering the bladder. (Hinman, 1993) The vas deferens crosses in front of the ureters while the ureters; pass in front of the end of the seminal vesicle in the male. Whereas, in the female, they lie behind the ovary and at the ischial spine are in close proximity with the suspensory ligament of the ovary. The ovarian vessels make an oblique crossing over the ureters as a potential vulnerable site for injury in gynecological operations. After entering the parametrium of the broad ligaments, they run through the uterosacral, cardinal and vesicouterine ligaments. Then, they cross the lateral and posterior parts of the uterine arteries. The left ureter crossing the uterine artery runs anteromedially about 1 cm above the lateral vaginal fornix and from 1 to 4 cm lateral to the cervix passes through the anterior aspect of the vagina before entering the bladder. Thus, ureter is mostly injured as it crosses inferior to the uterine artery. (Elliot & McAninch, 2006)

The blood supply of the ureter is so remarkable with multiple arteries anastomosing along its length. Thus, the division of any of the ureteral arteries does not usually produce ischemia. (Anderson et.al, 2007) The proximal ureteral arteries most often are supplied by the renal arteries (30%). The aorta provides 15% and the gonadal arteries 8% of its blood supply. Distally, the superior (12%) and inferior (12%) vesical arteries and internal iliac arteries (9%) provide the arterial supply to the lower portion of the ureter. (Hinman, 1993) The uretero-subperitoneal arteries lie outside the ureteral sheath. At the ureteral wall the arteries divide into "ureteral" arteries supplying the periureteral arterial plexus and the "subperitoneal" arteries supplying the periureteral tissue. (Landman & Pattaras, 2005) It is important to know that; the blood supply of the ureter in the abdomen is medial, while in the pelvis the blood supply is lateral. The ureteral arteries divide on the entering the loose ureteral sheath into long ascending and descending branches. Whereas; the subperitoneal arteries supply the periureteral tissue and provide a distribution to the peritoneum. Venules are distributed as a delicate network throughout the ureteral adventitia. The proximal ureter is drained via small veins into the renal or gonadal veins whereas; the distal end drain into those of broad ligament (in females), pelvic plexus and adjacent veins.

3. Patient selection and diagnostic work-up

Iatrogenic or traumatic injuries of the proximal 2/3 of the ureter, proximal ureteral stricture (e.g. due to stone, radiation, inflammation), retrocaval ureter (RCU) presenting with reduced ipsilateral kidney function or symptomatic, ureteral endometriosis, proximal ureteral obstruction (e.g: crossing vessels, neoplasia, aberrant ureteral position, valves), ureteral ectopia and some duplication anomalies of the urinary tract (e.g. functioning upper pole hydronephrosis without ureterocele) are the main indications of LUU. In most cases, a kind of imaging modality such as intravenous urography (IVP) or computerized tomography (CT) urography is needed to demonstrate the site of ureteric problem or intrinsic or extrinsic pathology leading to hydronephrosis. If these imaging modalities are inconclusive, a cystoscopy and retrograde or antegrade pyelography are useful for identifying pathological processes. For some cases having problems such as diminished vascular supply or concomitant infection that may impair wound healing leading to urinary extravasation after surgery, placement of nephrostomy tube is advocated. In those cases, the nephrostomy tube should be kept in place until ensuring the patency of the anastomosis.

Before surgery, the patient should undergo routine preoperative laboratory investigations, including total blood count, kidney function tests, and coagulation tests [such as, prothrombin time, partial thromboplastin time, and international normalized ratio (INR)]. Meanwhile, preoperative preparation of the patient should also include early withdrawal of drugs, such as acetylsalicylic acid or anticoagulants that affect platelet function. It is worth mentioning that, chronic renal failure or receiving hemodialysis treatment is not contraindications for laparoscopic ureteric reconstruction. (Sanli et al., 2010)

4. Preoperative auxiliary instrumentation

Laparoscopic ureteroureterostomy can be performed with transperitoneal (TP) or retroperitoneal (RP) approaches. Whether TP or RP approach is being used, it may be time saving to insert preoperatively a double-J (DJ) stent in low dorsal lithotomy position. In case of strictures or obstruction in the ureteral segment where the DJ stent cannot be inserted, it is advised to leave a ureteral stent as much as closed to the obstruction with its tether secured to the glans penis in males or the ipsilateral groin in females. This method will probably ease finding of pathological ureteral segment especially in cases of severe fibrosis. In addition, it is generally advocated to receive a clear liquid diet for 24 hours and a rectal suppository a night before the procedure.

5. Laparocopic ureteroureterostomy - Surgical technique

The principles of laparoscopic ureteric reconstruction are not different from those established for open surgery. These are ensuring good vascular supply in both ureteric ends with care to preserve the adventitia, complete excision of pathological lesions or nonviable tissue to a bleeding edge, good drainage with stenting and a wide spatulated and adequate ureteric end for tension-free anastomosis of mucosa to mucosa. (Elliot & McAninch, 2006; Png & Chapple, 2000)

5.1 Transperitoneal (TP) approach

After insertion of a Foley urethral catheter the patient is secured in a modified flank position over the kidney break at a 45-60° angle. A Veress needle is used to create a pneumoperitoneum and a 10-mm camera port is inserted at the level of umbilicus just lateral to the rectus abdominis muscle. On the occasion that the patient is slim; umbilicus may be used for this purpose. In right sided LUU, a 5-mm and a 10-mm port is inserted at the 1/3 caudal and 1/3 cranial points along a virtual line between xiphoid process and anterior superior iliac spine), respectively. Whereas, in case of left sided LUU, 5 and 10-mm port are inserted vice versa.

After proper port placement, the line of Toldt is incised and the colon is deflected medially to provide exposure of the RP (retroperitoneal) structures including inferior vena cava, ureter, gonadal vein, duodenum and renal pelvis in right side; ureter and gonadal vein in the left side. Subsequently, the ureter is found with proper RP dissection and problematic segment is visualized. This problematic ureter is then resected, making sure to reach healthy, well vascularized ureteral ends. If the situation is an injury due to thermal injury, wide debridement may be required because microvascular damage can extend for 2 cm beyond the evidence of visible injury. (Amato et al., 1970)

5.2 Retroperitoneal approach

For RP approach, the patient is placed in full lateral decubitus position with overextension in order to increase the distance between the ports. For port position, an incision is made below the 12th rib in the posterior axillary line for 10-mm camera port and after division of muscular layer and lumbodorsal fascia RP space is entered and dilated with a balloon dissector. A 5-mm trocar is inserted below the costal margin in the anterior axillary line and another 10-mm trocar is inserted 2 cm above the superior border of iliac crest in the midaxillary line in right sided cases. Ten and 5-mm trocars are inserted vice versa in left sided cases.

5.3 Ureteroureterostomy technique

Spatulated ureteroureterostomy (UU) is the gold standard technique in patients with good vascular supply in both ureteric ends and adequeate ureteric length for tension-free anastomosis. If the lengths of proximal or distal ureter do not allow tension free anastomosis, kidney may be mobilized for gaining some extra length. Generally the following basic approach is applied: After adequate exposure, both upper and lower ureter is transected sharply and spatulated laterally and medially as needed. Spatulation helps the meticulous watertight suturing while preventing the rotation of the ureter. One of the essential roles of the spatulation process is the preservation of the longitudinal ascending and descending branches of the ureteral arteries as well as allows wider luminal diameter. It is accepted that the placement of stay sutures can improve one's ability to properly direct the incisions while minimizing trauma to the tissues. (Lucas & Sundaram, 2011) However, it should be noted that placing stay sutures may need extra trochars for making them functional. Instead of this 12 o'clock and 6 o'clock sutures may be used for this purpose (Figure 1 and 2). Thereupon, a tension-free watertight UU is fashioned (over a DJ stent) using posterior and anterior wall closures of interrupted or running stitches with absorbable suture materials such as 4-0 or 5-0 polyglactin/polydioxanone sutures. The authors of the present chapter prefer to use interrupted sutures which are not too close together (2-3 mm apart) to prevent ischemia of the suture line.

Before completion of the reconstruction, if not inserted before, a DJ stent is placed to secure the anastomosis (Figure 3 and 4). However, one should be ensured that proximal end of the stent is in the renal pelvis; while distal end in the bladder. The proximal end of the stent may be visualized in the proximal uterer or renal pelvis but sometimes it may be difficult to observe the distal end if it is in the bladder. For confirming this issue, the bladder may be filled with methylene blue via the urethral catheter and observe reflux of blue urine through the stent. At the last occasion, cystoscopy may be performed to see the stent within the bladder. For securing the anastomosis and facilitate wound healing, repaired ureteral segment may be wrapped with an omental flep in transperitoneal approach. Subsequently, if placed stay sutures are released and haemostasis is checked with lowering the pressure of pneumo- or pneumoretroperitoneum to 4 mmHg. Eventually, a drain is positioned over the renal fossa and left overnight with a Foley urethral catheter. For injuries at or below the pelvic brim, ureteroneocystostomy should be the treatment of choice which is beyond the scope of this chapter.

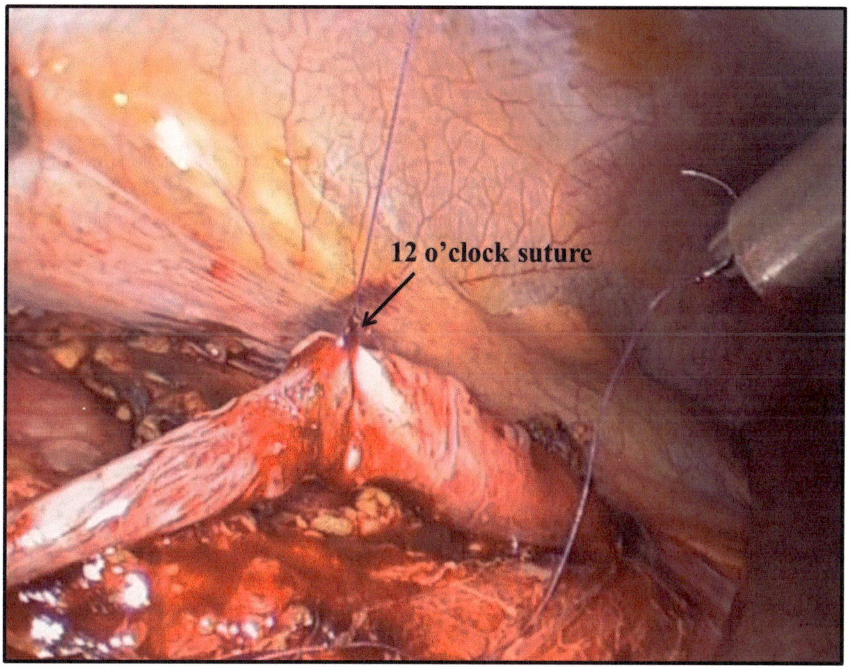

Fig. 1. "12 o'clock suture" is used as stay suture that helps direct visualization and minimizing trauma to surrounding tissues

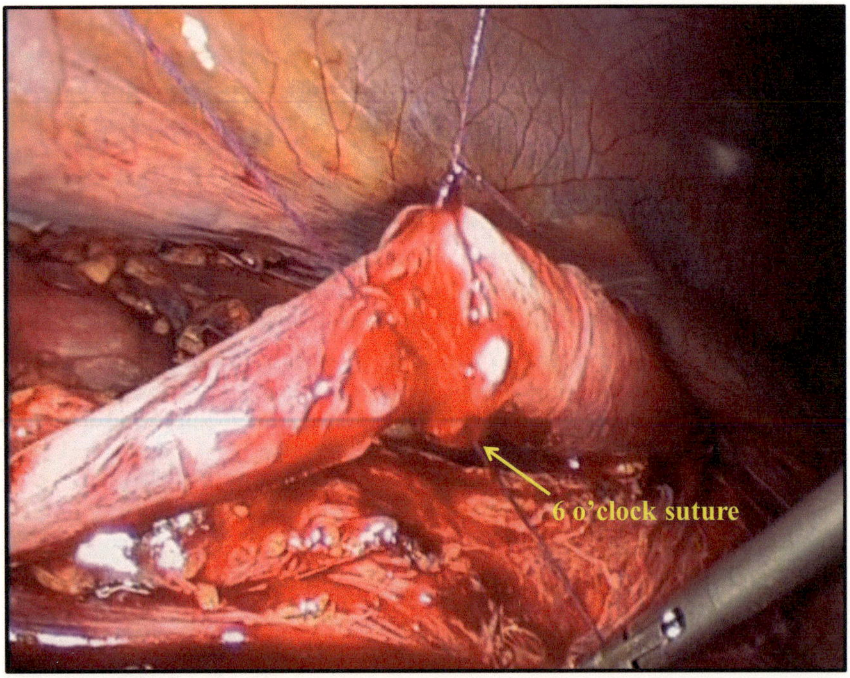

Fig. 2. “6 o'clock suture” helps completion of anterior and posterior closure of anastomosis separately

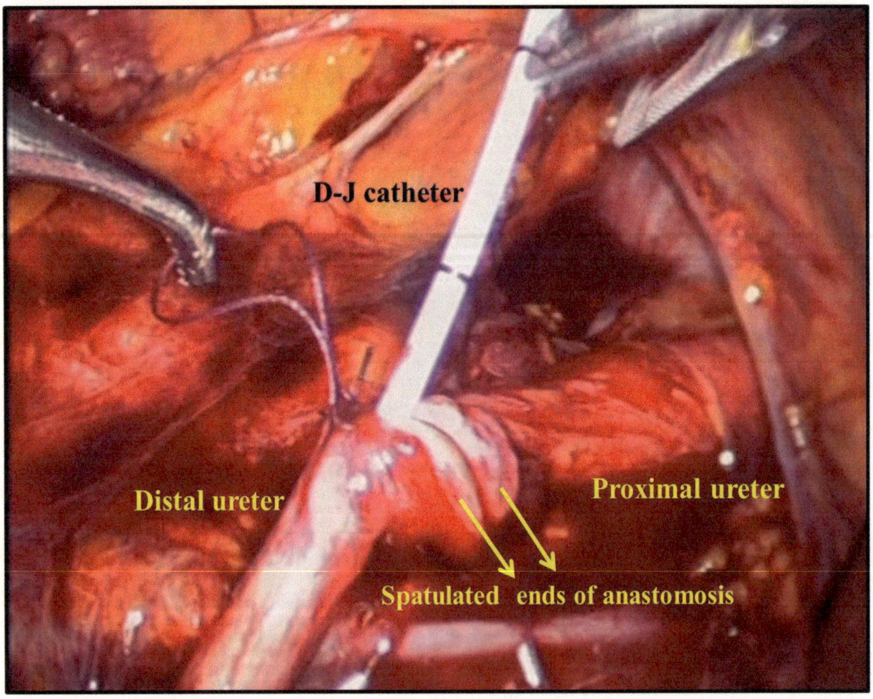

Fig. 3. Double J catheter insertion through anterior wall of anastomosis

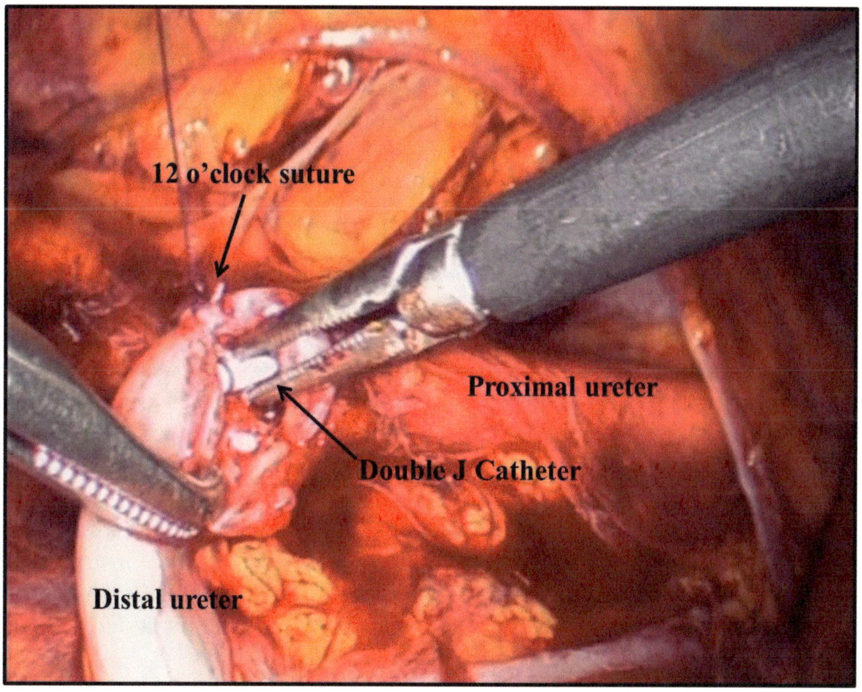

Fig. 4. Double J catheter inserted into renal pelvis

6. Transuretero-ureterostomy technique

Before Hendren popularized transuretero-ureterostomy (TUU) for use in undiversion, the technique has been restricted to patients who had suffered trauma or disease to the distal ureter, the excision of which left a defect that was too long to be bridged by mobilizing the bladder upwards by any means. (Hendren, 1973; Hodges et al., 1963) Other indications of TUU are cystectomy and substitution cystoplasty, Mitrofanoff-type urinary diversion and failed urinary diversion. (Kaiho et al., 2011; Noble et al., 1997) In 1999, Dechet et al. demonstrated the feasibility of laparoscopic TUU in a porcine model. (Dechet et al., 1999) Piaggio and Gonzalez first reported successful laparoscopic TUU in 3 children with ureteral obstruction, refluxing megaureter and ureteral injury after bladder diverticulectomy. (Piaggio & Gonzalez, 2007) The basic principles in open TUU are valid for the laparoscopic surgery, as well. These are mobilizing the ureter to be transposed across the posterior abdominal wall above the point of origin of the inferior mesenteric artery (to avoid kinking), to mobilize the recipient ureter to reduce the tension and to use an appropriate caliber stent across anastomosis. (Noble et al., 1997) For anastomosis, a small elliptic portion is excided from the medial wall of the recipient ureter and after spatulation of the donor ureter, an end to side anastomosis is performed. (Pesce et al, 2001) Although transureteroureterostomy has been proved to be safe and effective procedure, its place should certainly be restricted to ureteric defects above the pelvic brim, where a ureteroneocystostomy is not possible. (Png & Chapple, 2000) Transuretero-ureterostomy is a challenging approach used in selective cases; laparoscopic TUU is even more arduous because of the difficulty of passing donor ureter under mesocolon to the recipient ureter and currently should be reserved for very experienced referral centers. It is worth mentioning that inadequate surgical technique leading to urine leakage and subsequent stricture may compromise the drainage of the patent system. This is also valid for donor ureters with compromised vasculature due to radiation treatment or periureteral infection. Meanwhile TUU is discouraged if the renal unit on the side of injured ureter has minimal function.

7. Post-operative care and follow-up

In case of doubt, a plain abdominal film may be obtained to confirm the stent position. Since ureteral reconstruction generally leads to clean-contaminated wound, prophylaxis with 2nd generation cephalosporins is suggested. (Grabe et al, 2011) However, in case of positive urine culture before surgery, suitable antibiotics according to urine culture should be continued at least 7-10 days. The DJ stent should be removed in 2-6 weeks postoperatively. Retrograde pyelography (RGP) is not necessary while removing DJ catheter. We do not advocate DJ stents with an externalized tether since they may be a source of urinary tract infection (UTI). An IVP obtained 3 months after the operation can demonstrate the patency of anastomosis and is an excellent follow-up modality to discover any problems in continuity of urinary tract. The IVP can also demonstrate strictures and irregularities of reconstructed ureter. In case of any patency suspicion a 3-dimention reconstruction of a CT or magnetic resonance (MR) urography can facile the diagnosis. Six, 12 month and thereafter yearly follow up with IVP and yearly renal ultrasonography is recommended for 3 years.

8. Associated complications

Urinary tract infection, bleeding, haematoma formation, prolonged urine leakage from the drain and concomitant ileus (in TP approach) are the early complications that can be encountered with LUU. Meanwhile urinoma formation, retroperitoneal abscess and peritonitis may occur. The rate of early complications was found to be 3.8% (n= 4) in 109 renal units with the evaluation of the current literature (Table 1-4)

Urinary tract infection can be managed with administration of antibiotics; the bleeding may require re-exploration, whereas haematoma can be followed with serial haematocrit counts and ultrasonography. Prolonged leakage from the drain and ileus due to urinary leakage may require replacement of DJ stent under fluoroscopic control or nephrostomy tube placement.

Ureteral stricture, fistulae formation, undrained urinoma formation and periureteral abscess are the late complications that may require re-exploration and anastomosis revision. The rate of late complications was found to be 2.8% (n= 3, Table 1-4) in 109 renal units mentioned in the literature.

9. Outcomes analysis

In 1949 Anderson and Hynes published the first case of UU for retrocaval ureter. (Anderson & Hynes, 1949) Currently, open ureteric reconstruction is the standard of care. LUU has been successfully used for surgical correction of reterocaval ureters (RCU) since 1994. (Baba et al., 1994)

Retrocaval ureter is a rare congenital abnormality (incidence of 1 in 1000) that results in external ureteral compression by the inferior vena cava (IVC) and becomes symptomatic in the 3rd or 4th decade of life. Its etiology is presumed to be abnormal embryologic

Author	*Baba* 1994	*Polascik* 1998	*Salomon* 1999	*Mugiya* 1999	*Ameda* 2001	*Gupta* 2001	*Ramalingam* 2003	*T-Machado* 2005#	*Xu* 2008	*Singh* 2010*	*Li* 2010	*Autorino* 2010	*Sanli* 2010
Indication	RCU	RCU	RCU	RCU	RCU	RCU	RCU	RCU	RCU	RCU	RCU	RCU	RCU
Approach	Trans.	Trans.	Retro	Retro	Trans/Retro	Retro	Trans	Retro	Retro	Trans	Retro	Trans	Trans.
Method	Traditional	Traditional	Traditional	Traditional	Traditional	Traditional	Traditional	Traditional	Traditional	Traditional	Traditional	Single site	Traditional
No of cases	1	1	1	1	1/1	1	2	1	7	1	10	1	3
Mean Operative Time (min.)	570	225	270	300	450/400	210	225	130	128.6	120	82	180	118
Anastomosis Time (min.)	150	45	NA	NA	NA	NA	NA	40	36	NA	NA	NA	38,3
Anastomosis Technique	Interrupted	Interrupted	Interrupted	Running	Interrupted	Interrupted	Interrupted	Running	Interrupted	NA	Interrupted+ running	Running	Interrupted
No of Ports	5	3	4	4	4/4	3	4	3	3	4	3	Single port	3
Estimated Blood Loss (ml)	NA	NA	<20	50	<20	NA	Insignificant	50	20 (15-50)	NA	< 10	NA	76
Ureteral stent placement	NA	Preop.	NA	Preop.	Preop.	NA	NA	NA	NA	NA	NA	NA	Preop./none
Double J Placement	Intarop.	Intraop.	Preop.	Intraop	Intraop.	Preop.	Preop	Intraop.	Intraop.	Intraop.	Intraop.	Preop.	Preop/Intraop
Foley removal (days)	NA	2	NA	NA	NA	NA	NA	NA	5-7	NA	2	1	2.6
Drain removal (days)	NA	NA	2	5	1/1	2	3	NA	NA	2	NA	2	2.6
Hospital Stay (days)	9	4	7	NA	NA	3	4.5	2	6.5 (5-9)	3	6.5	2	3.3
DJ removal (weeks)	NA	4	4	12	4/4	6	8	6	4-6	4	4-6	4	4
Follow up (months)	NA	4	6	6	NA	3	7	3	16	4	52	3	4,3
Recovery	uneventful	uneventful	Uneventful	Uneventful	uneventful	uneventful	uneventful	uneventful	uneventful	uneventful	uneventful	uneventful	Uneventful
Complications													
Postoperative complications	none	none	none	None	None	None	1 (ileus)	none	None	none	none	none	None
Late on-set complications	none	None	none	none	None	None	none	none	none	none	None	none	none

Author suggested extracorporeal anostomosis to reach shorter operative time
*This report includes two case; ureteroureterostomy and pyelopyelostomy, only informations about ureteroureterostomy listed in this table.
NA: Not available

Table 1. Studies evaluating LUU for RCU.

Author	*Nezhat* 1992	*Nezhat* 1998	*Simforoosh* 2005	*Ou* 2005	*Cholkeri-Singh* 2007	*Simmons* 2007	*Carvalho* 2008	*Mereu* 2010
Indication	Endometriozis	Endometriosis	Transitional Cell Carcinoma	Stricture	Transected	Stricture	Stricture	Endometriosis
Approach	NA	NA	Trans.	Trans.	Trans.	Trans.	Trans.	Trans.
Method	Traditional	Traditional	Traditional	Traditional	Traditional	Traditional	Traditional	Traditional
No of patients	1	8	1	4	2	5	1	17
Mean Operative Time (min.)	187	NA	NA	100-240	NA	NA	NA	NA
Anastomosis Time (min.)	35	NA	NA	NA	NA	NA	NA	NA
Anastomosis Technique	Interrupted	NA	Running	Interrupted	Interrupted	NA	NA	Interrupted
No of Ports	NA	NA	3	5	3	4	4	4
Estimated Blood Loss (ml)	NA	<100	NA	NA	NA	86	NA	NA
Ureteral stent placement	NA	NA	NA	Preop.	Preop.	NA	Preop.	NA
Double J Placement	Preop.	NA	Intraop.	Preop.	Intraop.	Intraop.	Intraop.	Intraop.
Foley removal (days)	1	NA	NA	NA	6	NA	8	NA
Drain removal (days)	1	NA	NA	NA	4.5	5-7	12	NA
Hospital Stay (days)	2	NA	3	1.5	3	3	NA	NA
DJ removal (weeks)	6	NA	NA	6	6	4-6	6	NA
Follow up (months)	3	24	9	12	5	24	6	NA
Recovery	Uneventful	Uneventful	Uneventful	Uneventful	Uneventful	Uneventful	Uneventful	Uneventful
Complications								
Postoperative complications	None	None	None	None	None	None	None	none
Late on-set complications	None	1 (stricture)	None	none	none	None	none	2 (stricture)

NA: Not available

Table 2. Studies evaluating LUU for different indications.

Author	*Bhandarkar* 2005	*Nagraj* 2006	*Gonzalez* 2006	*Kutikov* 2007#	*Piaggio* 2007&	*Steyaert* 2009	*Storm* 2010
Indication	Congenital midureteral stricture	Retrocaval Ureter	Duplicated ureter	Duplicated ureter	Different etiologies∞	Duplicated ureter	Duplicated ureter
Approach	Trans.	Trans.	Trans.	Trans.	Trans.	Trans.	Trans.
Method	Traditional	Traditional	Traditional	Traditional	Traditional	Traditional	Traditional
No of patients	4	1	6 (8 operation)	3	3	2	7
Mean Operative Time (min.)	NA	100	257	186	263,6	120	187
Anastomosis Time (min.)	NA	NA	NA	NA	NA	NA	NA
Anastomosis Technique	Interrupted	NA	Interrupted+running	Running	Running	Running	Interrupted+Running
No of Ports	3	3	3-4*	3	4	4	3
Estimated Blood Loss (ml)	NA	NA	2.7	NA	47	NA	Minimal
Ureteral stent placement	Preop.	NA	Preop.	Preop.	Preop.	Preop.	Preop.
Double J Placement	Preop.	Intraop.	Intraop.	Intraop.	Preop.	NA	Preop.
Foley removal (days)	2	NA	1.5	NA	1-2	2.5	2
Drain removal (days)	2	2	2	NA	1-2	2	No drain
Hospital Stay (days)	4	3	3	2.25	3.33	5.5	2
DJ removal (weeks)	6	2	3	6	2-4	1	4-6
Follow up (months)	18	2	10.7	3	6	6	8
Recovery	Uneventful	Uneventful	Uneventful	Uneventful	uneventful	Uneventful	Uneventful
Complications							
Postoperative complications	None	None	2 (febril UTI)	none	1 (urine leakage)$	None	None
Late on-set complications	none	none	none	None	none	None	none

* Three ports for unilateral, four ports for bilateral duplication
#This report includes three laparoscopic ureteroureterostomies, two robot-assisted laparoscopic ureteroureterostomy and one laparoscopic Scardino-Prince flap. Table only lists three laparoscopic ureteroureterostomies
&Consists of laparoscopic transureteroureterostomies
∞Unilateral ureteral obstruction after cross-trigonal reimplantation for vesicoureteral reflux, unilateral refluxing megaureter and ureteral injury after bladder diverticulectomy
$Spontaneously resolved in less than 24 hours
NA: Not available

Table 3. Studies evaluating LUU performed for diffent indications in pediatric urology.

Author	*Yee* 2006	*Mufarrij* 2007	*Hemal* 2008	*Passerotti* 2008	*Lee* 2009	*Smith* 2009
Indication	Obstructed upper pole with renal ectopia	Stricture	Retrocaal ureter	Midureteral stricture*	Stricture-Transection	Pediatric; RCU,crossing vessels
Approach	Trans.	Trans.	Trans.	Trans.	Trans.	Trans.
Method	Robot-assisted	Robot-assisted	Robot-assisted	Robot-assisted	Robot-assisted	Robot-assisted
No of patients	1	2	1	3	3	2
Mean Operative Time (min.)	485	218.5	NA	244	136.6	283.5
Anastomosis Time (min.)	NA	NA	NA	NA	NA	NA
Anastomosis Technique	Running	Running	Interrupted	Interrupted	Running	Running
No of Ports	4	4	4	4	4	4
Estimated Blood Loss (ml)	15	55	NA	21.7	NA	12.5
Ureteral stent placement	Preop.	Preop.	NA	NA	Preop.	NA
Double J Placement	Intraop.	Intraop.	Intraop.	Preop.	Intraop.	Preop.
Foley removal (days)	2	NA	1	NA	NA	1
Drain removal (days)	2	NA	1	NA	NA	1
Hospital Stay (days)	3	2.5	3	3.5	3	1
DJ removal (weeks)	4	NA	6	NA	6	½
Follow up (months)	3	12.5	3	11.6	24	1
Recovery	Uneventful	Uneventful	Uneventful	Uneventful	Uneventful	Uneventful
Complications						
Postoperative complications	None	None	None	None	None	None
Late on-set complications	none	None	none	None	None	none

*ureteral valve, an inflammatory response with polyarteritis nodosa, an ureteral stone associated stricture

NA: Not available

Table 4. LUU'ies performed with robotic technology.

development of the IVC, which results from the major portion of the infrarenal IVC being formed from the subcardinal vein that lies ventral to the ureter. (Considine, 1966) For the first time, Baba et al performed a TP approach in a case of RCU with mean operative time (OT) of 570 min. and an interrupted anastomosis in 150 min. (Baba et al., 1994) A decade was needed to shorten the OT to 82 min. reported by Li et al. (Li et al., 2010) Ten cases in the literature were performed through the TP approach with a mean OT of 235 min., whereas 22 cases with a RP approach having mean OT of 138 min do exist (Table 1). Even though the OT in RP approach is shorter, retroperitoneoscopy has its own disadvantage of limited working space for laparoscopic manipulation. On the contrary, the advantage of RP approach is the rapid and direct access to renal pelvis and ureter without violating the peritoneal cavity. (Li et al., 2010) Even if a decent number of authors claim that the RP-LUU is less time-consuming (Ameda et al., 2001; Gupta et al, 2001; Li et al., 2010; Mugiya et al., 1999; Salomon et al., 1999; Tobias-Machado et al., 2005; Xu et al., 2009); some prefer the TP access and affirm that it is easier than the RP approach. (Ameda et al., 2001; Autorino et al., 2010; Baba et al., 1994; Polascik & Chen, 1998; Ramalingam & Selvarajan, 2003; Sanli et al., 2010; Singh et al., 2010) Given the small number of cases reported in the literature, and bias from case selection; the OT favors the RP approach, nonetheless the surgeon should prefer the method that is most familiar with.

There is a general impression that performing an anastomosis with interrupted sutures is safer while performing UU. Most of the authors reporting LUU for RCU used interrupted suturing technique. (Ameda et al., 2001; Baba et al., 1994; Elliot & McAninch, 2006; Mugiya et al., 1999; Polascik & Chen, 1998; Ramalingam & Selvarajan, 2003; Salomon et al., 1999; Sanli et al., 2010; Xu et al., 2009) However, none of the authors using running sutures have reported any complication regarding urine anastomotic stricture. (Autorino et al., 2010; Li et al., 2010; Mugiya et al., 1999; Tobias-Machado et al., 2005) Li et al., has used posterior ureteroureteral anastomosis with running suture which every 2 sutures were coupled with a lock-stitch suture and anterior interrupted suture anastomosis. This technique reduced their OT to a mean of 82 min without compromising the anastomosis. Meanwhile, some authors advocate performing pyelopyelostomy instead of UU; because it is less likely to produce stricture formation due to the larger caliber structures as well as better blood supply in the level of renal pelvis. (Bhandarkar et al., 2003; Dogan et al., 2010; Simforoosh et al., 2005) We believe that this technique is a rational option especially for patients with Type I retrocaval ureter which is characterized by S or fish-hook deformity of the ureter and is usually associated with moderate to severe hydronephrosis (Type II RCU is sickle-cell shaped and is associated with mild hydronephrosis). In addition, pyelopyelostomy with the preservation of retrocaval segment was suggested by Simforoosh et al. (Simforoosh et al., 2005) The authors' rationale for leaving the retrocaval segment was the dysplastic and narrow nature of this segment which may not be suitable for UU. Meanwhile, leaving this segment may also prevent some complications such as venous bleeding during dissection of vena cava.

Meanwhile, some authors placed a ureteral stent preoperatively and insert a DJ catheter during the operation (Ameda et al., 2001; Baba et al., 1994; Li et al., 2010; Mugiya et al., 1999; Polascik & Chen, 1998; Sanli et al., 2010; Singh et al., 2010; Tobias-Machado et al., 2005; Xu et al., 2009) Others, insert preoperatively a DJ stent and postulate that lessens OT. (Autorino et al., 2010; Gupta et al., 2001; Ramalingam & Selvarajan, 2003; Salomon et al., 1999; Sanli et al.,

2010) As mentioned before, we believe that placement of a DJ catheter before the operation is time saving.

In order to decrease the OT different approaches have been utilized. Tobias-Machado et al performed the anastomosis extracorporeally. (Tobias-Machado, 2005) The ureteral ends were exteriorized though the incision of the 12-mm port after enlarging the skin incision to 20-mm. Despite decreasing the OT, we believe that exteriorizing the ureteral ends require additional dissection of the ureters which may impair the ureteral blood supply. Meanwhile, a half open (extracorporeal) technique does not address and fit the rationale laparoscopy. Nevertheless, it may be rational to suggest the use of this technique to novice laparoscopists with limited dexterity for intracorporeal suturing.

Ureteral strictures (US) due to ureteral trauma, inflammation, stones or radiation are the leading indications for UU. Although, trauma to the ureter is relatively rare and accounts for only %1 of all urinary tract trauma, 75% of ureteric trauma is iatrogenic and of these 73%, 14% and %14 are in gynecological, urological and general surgical in origin, respectively. (Dobrowolski et al., 2002; Lynch et al., 2005) There is a trend of increase in incidence of iatrogenic urological trauma from 1990's due to development of new techniques such as ureteroscopy and laparoscopy. Ureteroscopy results in ureteral perforation in 2-6% of cases which is a significant risk factor for ureteral stricture. (Elliot & McAninch, 2006) LUU should be considered in patients with unsuccessful attempts by using standard minimal invasive therapies such as balloon dilatation and endoureterotomy with laser or electrocautery. While repairing the stricture, the length of the stricture has always been a subject of debate achieving tension-free anastomosis. Ou et al. published 3 cases of LUU performed on patients with US having operated for laparoscopic hysterectomy. (Ou et al., 2005) They have trimmed the necrotic tissue on ureteral ends, performed tension free LUU over DJ catheter and wrapped the repair with omentum. The authors suggested using LUU; when the injury is not close to the bladder and involves less than 1.5 cm of the ureter. They probably mentioned the use of this technique in strictures less than 1.5cm based on their clinical experience; but we believe that depending on the tortuosity of the ureter, more lengthy strictures may be repaired with LUU. Since for open surgery, it is known that defects up to 3 cm can be repaired at once without tension. (Mayor & Zingg, 1976) Meanwhile, if the defect is larger, this tension may be reduced by mobilizing and straightening its pelvic part. Cholkeri-Singh et al. have published 2 cases of laparoscopic ureteral repair after ureteral injury during laparoscopic procedures. (Cholkeri-Singh et al., 2007; Table 2) Similarly, Carvalho et al have reported successful repair of ureteral injury after hernia repair by LUU. (Carvalho et al., 2008) Furthermore, Simmons et al published 5 cases of LUU after stricture. (Simmons et al., 2007) All these authors acknowledge that favorable laparoscopic approach is possible if performed with the assistance of experienced surgeons.

Despite very limited evidence in the literature, laparoscopic segmental ureterectomy was suggested as alternative to open segmental ureterectomy for low grade transitional cell carcinoma (TCC) of the proximal and mid ureter. (Simforoosh et al., 2005) However, while performing this operation, one should leave a 1 cm safety margin proximally and distally and frozen section analysis for the both ureteral ends is highly recommended. Meanwhile, it is worth mentioning that TCC is very prone to port site metastasis and every attempt should be made to prevent this undesirable and life-threatening complication.

Urologic endometriosis is another disease that may require UU. Despite of the fact that urinary tract involvement is uncommon (1-5%), it may cause obstruction of the ureter leading to hydronephrosis. (Jimenez et al., 2000) In this circumstance, surgical resection of the involved ureteral segment is a viable option because it removes the disease and surrounding fibrosis. The first case of LUU in the literature is reported by Nezhat et al. (Nezhat et al, 1992) In a recent study, Antonelli et al., reported the outcomes of 11 patients with ureteral endometriosis treated with surgical excision. (Antonelli et al., 2006) Among these patients, endometriosis was found to be deeply infiltrating the muscle layer in 4 (intrinsic endometriosis), whereas only adventitia or periureteral tissues were affected in 7 (extrinsic endometriosis) patients. The authors reported no complications regarding UU technique in 2 patients and mentioned that laparoscopic ureterolysis is a more suitable approach for minimal, extrinsic and non-obstructive ureteral involvement; whereas LUU is favorable for intrinsic disease. Meanwhile, Mereu et al reported 17 cases of ureteral endometriosis managed with LUU. (Mereu et al., 2010) Of this cohort, 2 patients had complications with strictures postoperatively. Thus, the authors advocate the complete ureteral excision of the tissue involved since the left endometriosis tissue may lead to recurrences. Similar convincing outcomes were also reported by Nezhat et al (Table 2; Nezhat et al., 1998)

Laparoscopic ureteroureterostomy may have place in some pediatric urological diseases mentioned in Table 3. Briefly, the OT and hospital stay ranges between 100 and 263 min. and 2 and 5.5 days, respectively. After a mean follow-up of 7.7 months, 3 complications were encountered for the operation of 23 renal units. These were febrile UTIs in 2 patients and urine leakage that was spontaneously resolved within 24 hours in 1 patient. (Bhandarkar et a.,2005; González & Piaggio, 2007; Nagraj et al., 2006; Piaggio & González, 2007; Steyaert et al., 2009; Storm et al., 2010)

10. Novel techniques

Tissue engineering has been applied experimentally for the reconstitution of several urologic tissues and organs, including ureter. (Atala, 2004) In one of these studies, Osman et al. have reported the replacement of 3cm segment ureteral defect by acellular tube matrix from canine decellularized ureters. However, ureteral replacement with this naïve bioscaffold was unsuccessful due to fibrosis. (Osman et al., 2004) Smith et al reported a small intestinal submucosa (SIS) allograft to bridge a 2 cm ureteral defect and noted that SIS graft was replaced with ureteral growth in 9 weeks. (Smith et al., 2002) Meanwhile Matsunuma et al. used decellularized matrix with cultured uroepithelial cells for tissue engineered ureter and showed that angiogenesis of this bioscaffold may be increased by seeded bone marrow derived mononuclear cells. (Matsunuma et al., 2006) Recently, a model of "omental bioreactor" for differentiation of engineered neoureter was recently introduced by Baumert et al. (Baumert et al., 2007) In this model bladder biopsies were taken and smooth muscle and urothelial cells were cultured. Then the cultured cells were seeded to small intestinal submucosa (SIS) matrix. Afterwards the cultured cells were wrapped by the omentum around a silicone drain to obtain neoureters. Thus, the authors obtained mature well differentiated multilayered urothelium. Consequently, although animal studies express promising results, the actual ureteral replacement with viable grafts has to wait the studies to mature further (Baumert et al., 2008)

Fibrin sealants are being used more and more in urology. It has been used for laparoscopic pyeloplasty, partial nephrectomy, ureteral injuries, closure of ureterotomies in stone surgery and occlusion of the distal ureter while performing distal ureterectomy with "pluck" technique for the treatment of upper urinary tract TCC. (Eden et al., 1997; Kouba et al., 2004; Mueller et al., 2005; Schultz & Christiansen, 1985) Moreover, a large volume urine leakage after renal cyst decortication was stopped with endoscopic retrograde fibrin glue injection and ureteral stent placement. (Chen et al., 2011) Meanwhile, there is some evidence in the literature that fibrin sealants promote wound healing and reinforce ureteral anastomosis. (Kumar et al., 2001) In animal model, it was shown that LUU made by fibrin glue without stay sutures produced better radiographic findings, flow characteristics and histology. (Wolf et al., 1997) Consequently, fibrin sealants may be used for further water-tightness of the anastomosis. In addition, the use of tissue sealants may reduce the number of sutures placed for anastomosis which may theoretically decrease suture line ischemia. (Detweiler et al., 1999)

Robotic technology has been increasingly used in urological procedures. It tends to replace conventional laparoscopic techniques in complex urologic surgeries and especially in reconstructive procedures. Some series of robotic UU has been published recently. (Hemal et al., 2008; Lee et al., 2010) Apart from the ergonomic advantages for the surgeon and technical benefits such as meticulous sharp dissection and precise spatulation of the ureter with the aid of wristed instruments and magnified 3D vision; this technology did not yet contribute significantly over laparoscopy. (Hemal et al., 2008) However, it is worth mentioning that intracorporeal suturing is much easier with robot which is probably the most important factor on OT. The cost and the lack of haptic feedback are the major disadvantages of robotic technology. Recently, Lee et al. reported 3 successful re-anastomosis of the ureter robotically (Lee et al., 2010). The mean operation time was 136.6 minutes and none of the patients developed recurrent stricture after a 24 months of follow-up. Meanwhile, Smith et al. reported successful robotic UU in 2 children with the length of hospital stay roughly 30 hours. (Smith et al., 2009) The authors reported resolution of hydronephrosis at 1 month follow-up imaging. To our knowledge, 10 renal units were operated with the robot for different indications. The OT is ranging from 136.6 min to 485 min and no complication were encountered after mean follow-up ranging 1 to 24 months (Table 4).

Laparoendoscopic single-site (LESS) surgery for UU is promising and the feasibility of the technique has been reported by Autorino et al. in a patient diagnosed with RCU. (Autorino et al., 2010)

11. Conclusions

Ureteroureterostomy has always been a challenging procedure in the history of urology. Surgical approaches for UU have steadily evolved over the last 50 years paralleling the introduction of new technologies.

In the past decade, laparoscopy has been increasingly utilized for a variety of complex urological procedures. The recent technological advancements in laparoscopy had significant impacts on urologic surgery. The technical refinement and development of laparoscopic devices have enabled laparoscopic surgeons perform challenging urinary tract reconstructions. Due to the small number of cases, LUU cannot be stated that it is superior to open surgery. But the benefit of magnification with improved visualization and minimal invasiveness provide meticulous dissection and precise approximation which renders the laparoscopic approach beneficial to open.

12. References

Amato JJ, Billy LJ, Gruber RP, et al. Vascular injuries. An experimental study of high and low velocity missile wounds. Arch surg 1970; 101: 167-174.

Ameda K, Kakizaki H, Harabayashi T, Watarai Y, Nonomura K, Koyanagi T. Laparoscopic ueteroureterostomy for retrocaval. Int J Urol. 2001; 8: 71-4.

Anderson JC, Hynes W. Retrocaval ureter; a case diagnosed pre-operatively and treated successfully by a plastic operation. Br J Urol. 1949;21:209-14.

Anderson JK, Kabalin JN, Caddedu JA. (2007) Surgical anatomy of the Retroperitoneum, Adrenals, Kidneys, and Ureters. In: Campbell-Walsh Urology, Wein AJ, Kavoussi LR, Novick AC, Partin AW, Peters CA, editors, p. 32-7. Philadelphia: Saunders;

Antonelli A, Simeone C, Zani D, Sacconi T, Minini G, Canossi E, Cucino SC. Clinical aspects and surgical treatment of urinary tract endometriosis: Our experience with 31 cases. Eur Urol 2006; 49: 1093-1098.

Atala A. Tissue engineering for the replacement of organ function in the genitourinary system. Am J Transplant. 2004;4 Suppl 6:58-73.

Autorino R, Khanna R, White MA, Haber GP, Shah G, Kaouk JH, Stein RJ. Laparoendoscopic single-site repair of retrocaval ureter: first case report. Urology. 2010;76:1501-5.

Baba S, Oya M, Miyahara M, Deguchi N, Tazaki H. Laparoscopic surgical correction of circumcaval ureter. Urology. 1994; 44: 122-6.

Baumert H, Mansouri D, Fromont G, et al. Terminal urothelium differentiation of engineered neoureter after in vivo maturation in the "omental bioreactor". Eur Urol 2007;52:1492–8.

Baumert H, Hekmati M, Dunia I, Mansouri D, Massoud W, Molinié V, Benedetti EL, Malavaud B. Laparoscopy in ureteral engineering: a feasibility study. Eur Urol. 2008;54:1154-63.

Bhandarkar DS, Lalmalani JG, Shivde S. Laparoscopic ureterolysis and reconstruction of a retrocaval ureter. Surg Endosc. 2003 17: 1851-1852.

Bhandarkar DS, Lalmalani JG, Shah VJ. Laparoscopic resection and ureteroureterostomy for congenital midureteral stricture. J Endourol. 2005;19:140-2.

Carvalho GL, Santos FG, Santana EF, Foinquinos RA, Passos GO Jr, Brandt CT, Lacerda CM. Laparoscopic repair of a ureter damaged during inguinal herniorrhaphy. Surg Laparosc Endosc Percutan Tech. 2008;18:526-9.

Chen ML, Tomaszewski JJ, Matoka DJ, Ost MC. Management of urine leak after laparoscopic cyst decortication with retrograde endoscopic fibrin glue application and ureteral stent placement.J Endourol. 2011;25:71-4.

Cholkeri-Singh A, Narepalem N, Miller CE. Laparoscopic ureteral injury and repair: case reviews and clinical update. J Minim Invasive Gynecol. 2007;14:356-61.

Considine J. Retrocaval ureter. A review of the literature with a report on two new cases followed for fifteen years and two years respectively. Br J Urol. 1966; 38: 412-2

Dechet CB, Young MM, Segura JW. Laparoscopic transureteroureterostomy: demonstration of its feasibility in swine. J Endourol 1999;13:487–93

Detweiler MB, Detweiler JG, Fenton J. Sutureless and reduced suture anastomosis of hollow vessels with fibrin glue: a review. J Invest Surg. 1999;12:245-62.

Dobrowolski Z, Kusionowicz J, Drewniak T, Habrat W, Lipczynski W, Jakubik P, Weglarz W. Renal and ureteric trauma: diagnosis and management in Poland. BJU Int 2002; 89: 748-751.

Dogan HS, Oktay B, Vuruskan H, Yavascaoglu I. Treatment of retrocaval ureter by pure laparoscopic pyelopyelostomy: experience on 4 patients. Urology 2010; 75: 1343-1347

Dunn MD, Portis AJ, Shalhav AL, et al. Laparoscopic versus open radical nephrectomy: a 9-year experience. J Urol. 2000;164: 1153–115.

Eden CG, Sultana SR, Murray KH, Carruthers RK. Extraperitoneal laparoscopic dismembered fibrin-glued pyeloplasty: medium-term results. Br J Urol. 1997;80:382-9.

Elliot SP, McAninch JW. Ureteral injuries: external and iatrogenic. Urol clin North am 2006; 33: 55-66

González R, Piaggio L. Initial experience with laparoscopic ipsilateral ureteroureterostomy in infants and children for duplication anomalies of the urinary tract. J Urol. 2007;177:2315-8.

Guillonneau B, Abbou C, Doublet JD, Gaston R, Janetchek G, Mandressi A, et al. A proposal for a 'European Scoring System for laparoscopic operations in Urology" Eur Urol 2001;40:2-6.

Gupta NP, Hemal AK, Singh I, Khaitan A. Retroperitoneoscopic ureterolysis and reconstruction of retrocaval ureter. J Endourol. 2001;15:291-3.

Hemal AK, Rao R, Sharma S, Clement RG. Pure robotic retrocaval ureter repair. Int Braz J Urol. 2008;34:734-8.

Hendren WH. Some alternatives to urinary diversion in children. J Urol. 1978;119:652-60.

Hinman F. Kidney, Ureter, and Adrenal Glands, In: Atlas of Urosurgical Anatomy. Philadelphia: W.B. Saunders; 1993. p. 284-9.

Hodges CV, Moore RJ, Lehman TH, Behnam AM. Clinical experiences with transureteroureterostomy. J Urol. 1963;90:552-62.

Jimenez RE, Tiguert R, Hurley P, An T, Grignon DJ, Lawrence D, Triest J. Unilateral hydronephrosis resulting from intraluminal obstruction of the ureter by adenosquamous endometrioid carcinoma arising from disseminated endometriosis. Urology 2000; 1; 56: 331.

Kaiho Y, Ito A, Numahata K, Ishidoya S, Arai Y. Retroperitoneoscopic transureteroureterostomy with cutaneous ureterostomy to salvage failed ileal conduit urinary diversion. Eur Urol 2011; 59: 875-8

Kouba E, Tornehl C, Lavelle J, Wallen E, Pruthi RS. Partial nephrectomy with fibrin glue repair: measurement of vascular and pelvicaliceal hydrodynamic bond integrity in a live and abbatoir porcine model. J Urol. 2004;172:326-30.

Kumar U, Dickerson A, Sakamoto K, Albala DM, Turk TM. Effects of fibrin glue on injured rabbit ureter. J Endourol. 2001 Mar;15(2):205-7.

Kutikov A, Nguyen M, Guzzo T, Canter D, Casale P. Laparoscopic and robotic complex upper-tract reconstruction in children with a duplex collecting system. J Endourol. 2007;21:621-4.

Landman J, Pattaras JG. Urologic laparoscopic anatomy. In: Moore RG, Bishoff JT, Loening S, Docimo SG, editors. Minimally Invasive Surgery, London and New York: Taylor & Francis, 2005. P. 11-28.

Lee DI, Schwab CW, Harris A. Robot-assisted ureteroureterostomy in the adult: initial clinical series. Urology. 2010; 75: 570-573.

Li HZ, Ma X, Qi L, Shi TP, Wang BJ, Zhang X. Retroperitoneal laparoscopic ureteroureterostomy for retrocaval ureter: report of 10 cases and literature review. Urology. 2010; 76: 873-6

Lucas SM, Sundaram CP. Transperitoneal robot-assisted laparoscopic pyeloplasty. J Endourol. 2011;25:167-72.

Lynch TH, Lynch TH, Martínez-Piñeiro L, Plas E, Serafetinides E, Türkeri L, Santucci RA, Hohenfellner M; European Association of Urology, EAU Guidelines on urological trauma. Eur Uro 2005; 47,1-15.

Matsunuma H, Kagami H, Narita Y et al. Constructing a tissue-engineered ureter using a decellularized matrix with cultured uroepithelial cells and bone marrow-derived mononuclear cells. Tissue Eng. 2006; 12: 509–18.

Mayor G, Zingg EJ. Ureteroureteral anostomosis: In Urologic Surgery Diagnosis, Techniques and Postoperative Treatment. Stuttgart: Georg Thieme Publishers; 1976. p 284-289

Mereu L, Gagliardi ML, Clarizia R, Mainardi P, Landi S, Minelli L. Laparoscopic management of ureteral endometriosis in case of moderate-severe hydroureteronephrosis. Fertile Steril 2010; 93: 46-51.

M. Grabe, T.E. Bjerklund-Johansen, H. Botto, B. Wullt, M. Çek, K.G. Naber, R.S. Pickard, P. Tenke, F. Wagenlehner. Urological Infections EAU Guidelines 2011; DOI: 978-90-79754-96-0

Mueller TJ, DaJusta DG, Cha DY, Kim IY, Ankem MK. Ureteral fibrin sealant injection of the distal ureter during laparoscopic nephroureterectomy--a novel and simple modification of the pluck technique. Urology. 2010;75:187-92.

Mugiya S, Suzuki K, Ohhira T, Un-No T, Takayama T, Fujita K. Retroperitoneoscopic treatment of a retrocaval ureter. Int J Urol. 1999;6:419-22.

Nagraj HK, Kishore TA, Nagalakshmi S. Transperitoneal laparoscopic approach for retrocaval ureter. J Minim Access Surg. 2006;2:81-2.

Nezhat C, Nezhat F, Green B. Laparoscopic treatment of obstructed ureter due to endometriosis by resection and ureteroureterostomy: a case report. J Urol 1992 148: 865-868.

Nezhat CH, Nezhat F, Seidman D, Nezhat C. Laparosocopic ureteroureterostomy: a prospective follow-up of 9 patients. Prim Care Update Ob Gyns 1998; 5, 200.

Noble IG, Lee KT, Mundy AR. Transuretero-ureterostomy: a review of 253 cases. Br J Urol. 1997; 79 :20-3.

Osman Y, Shokeir A, Gabr M, El-Tabey N, Mohsen T, El-Baz M. Canine ureteral replacement with long acellular matrix tube: is it clinically applicable? J. Urol. 2004; 172: 1151–4.

Ou CS, Huang IA, Rowbotham R. Laparoscopic ureteroureteral anastomosis for repair of ureteral injury involving stricture.Int Urogynecol J Pelvic Floor Dysfunct. 2005; 16: 155-157

Piaggio LA, Gonzalez R. Laparoscopic transureteroureterostomy: a novel approach. J Urol 2007; 177: 2311–4.

Pesce C, Costa L, Campobasso P, Fabbro MA, Musi L. Successful use of transureteroureterostomy in children: a clinical study. Eur J Pediatr Surg. 2001; 11: 395-8.

Pereira BMT, Ogilvie MP, Gomez-Rodriguez JC, Ryan ML, Pena D, Marttos AC, Pizano LR, McKenney MG. A review of ureteral injuries after external trauma. Scand J Trauma Resusc Emerg Med 2010;18: 6

Piaggio LA, González R. Laparoscopic transureteroureterostomy: a novel approach. J Urol. 2007;177:2311-4.

Png JC, Chapple CR. Principles of ureteric reconstruction. Curr Opin Urol. 2000 May;10(3):207-12.

Polascik TJ, Chen RN. Laparoscopic ureteroureterostomy for retrocaval ureter. J Urol. 1998;160:121-2.

Ramalingam M, Selvarajan K. Laparoscopic transperitoneal repair of retrocaval ureter: report of two cases. J Endourol. 2003;17:85-7.

Salomon L, Hoznek A, Balian C, Gasman D, Chopin DK, Abbou CC.Retroperitoneal laparoscopy of a retrocaval ureter. BJU Int. 1999; 84: 181-2.

Sanli O, Onol FF, Tefik T, Simsek A, Naghiyev A, Onol SY. Transperitoneal laparoscopic ureteroureterostomy for the treatment of retrocaval ureter: analysis of 3 consecutive cases Turkish Journal of Urology 2010; 36: 309-313.

Sanli O, Tefik T, Ortac M, Karadeniz M, Oktar T, Nane I, Tunc M. Laparoscopic nephrectomy in patients undergoing hemodialysis treatment. JSLS. 2010;14:534-40

Schultz A, Christiansen LA. Fibrin adhesive sealing of ureter after ureteral stone surgery. A controlled clinical trial. Eur Urol. 1985;11:267-8.

Simforoosh N, Mosapour E, Maghsudi R. Laparoscopic ureteral resection and anastomosis for management of low-grade transitional-cell carcinoma. J Endourol. 2005;19:287-9.

Simforoosh N, Nouri-Mahdavi K, Tabibi A. Laparoscopic pyelopyelostomy for retrocaval segment: first report of 6 cases. J Urol 2006; 175: 2166-2169.

Simmons MN, Gill IS, Fergany AF, Kaouk JH, Desai MM. Laparoscopic ureteral reconstruction for benign stricture disease. Urology 2007;69:280-4.

Singh O, Gupta SS, Hastir A, Arvind NK. Laparoscopic transperitoneal pyelopyelostomy and ureteroureterostomy of retrocaval ureter: Report of two cases and review of the literature. J Minim Access Surg. 2010;6:53-5.

Smith TG III, Gettman M, Lindberg G, Napper C, Pearle MS, Cadeddu JA. Ureteral replacement using porcine small intestine submucosa in a porcine model. Urology 2002; 60: 931–4.

Smith KM, Shrivastava D, Ravish IR, Nerli RB, Shukla AR. Robot-assisted laparoscopic ureteroureterostomy for proximal ureteral obstructions in children. J Pediatr Urol 2009; 5: 475-479.

Steyaert H, Lauron J, Merrot T, Leculee R, Valla JS. Functional ectopic ureter in case of ureteric duplication in children: initial experience with laparoscopic low transperitoneal ureteroureterostomy. J Laparoendosc Adv Surg Tech A. 2009;19 Suppl 1:S245-7.

Storm DW, Modi A, Jayanthi VR. Laparoscopic ipsilateral ureteroureterostomy in the management of ureteral ectopia in infants and children. J Pediatr Urol. 2010 doi:10.1016/j.jpurol.2010.08.004

Tobias-Machado M, Lasmar MT, Wroclawski ER. Retroperitoneoscopic surgery with extracorporeal uretero-ureteral anastomosis for treating retrocaval ureter. Int Braz J Urol. 2005;31:147-50.

Wolf JS Jr, Soble JJ, Nakada SY, Rayala HJ, Humphrey PA, Clayman RV, Poppas DP. Comparison of fibrin glue, laser weld, and mechanical suturing device for the laparoscopic closure of ureterotomy in a porcine model.J Urol. 1997;157:1487-92.

Xu DF, Yao YC, Ren JZ, Liu YS, Gao Y, Che JP, Cui XG, Chen M. Retroperitoneal laparoscopic ureteroureterostomy for retrocaval ureter: report of 7 cases. Urology. 2009;74:1242-5.

Part 3

Latest Techniques

6

Navigated Ultrasound in Laparoscopic Surgery

Thomas Langø[1], Toril N. Hernes[1,2] and Ronald Mårvik[3]
[1]*SINTEF, Dept. Medical Technology,*
[2]*Norwegian University of Science and Technology (NTNU),*
[3]*National Center for Advanced Laparoscopic Surgery, St. Olavs Hospital,*
Norway

1. Introduction

Open surgery is the gold standard for abdominal surgeries. But over the last few decades, there has been an increasing demand to shift from open surgery to a minimally invasive approach to make the intervention and the post-operative phase less traumatizing for the patient. Advantages of laparoscopic surgery include decreased morbidity, reduced costs for society (less hospital time and quicker recovery), and also improved long-term outcomes when compared to open surgery. During laparoscopy, the surgeons make use of a video camera for instrument guidance. However, the video laparoscope can only provide two-dimensional (2D) surface visualization of the abdominal cavity. Laparoscopic ultrasound (LUS) provides information beyond the surface of the organs, and was therefore introduced by Yamakawa and coworkers in 1958 (Yamakawa et al., 1958). In 1991, Jakimowicz and Reuers introduced LUS scanning for examination of the biliary tree during laparoscopic cholecystectomy (Jakimowicz & Ruers, 1991). It seemed that LUS gave valuable information and has since expanded in use with the increase in laparoscopic procedures. LUS is today applied in laparoscopy in numerous ways for screening, diagnostics and therapeutic purposes (Jakimowicz, 2006; Richardson et al., 2010). Some examples of use are screening, like stone detection or identification of lymph nodes, diagnostic, like staging of disease or assessment of operability and resection range, and therauptic, like resection guidance or guidance of radio frequency and cryoablation. Harms and coworkers were the first to integrate an electromagnetic (EM) tracking sensor into the tip of a conventional laparoscopic ultrasound probe (Harms et al., 2001) and this made it possible to combine LUS with navigation technology, solving some of the orientation problems experienced when using laparoscopic ultrasound. The combination of navigation technology and LUS is becoming an active field of research to further improve the safety, accuracy, and outcome of laparoscopic surgery.

Navigation is the combined use of tracking and imaging technology to provide a visualization of the position of the tip of a surgical instrument relative to a target and surrounding anatomy. Various display and visualizations methods of both instruments and the medical images can be used. Preoperative images are useful for planning as well as for guidance during the initial phase of the procedure as long as the target area is in the retroperitoneum (Mårvik et al., 2004). When preoperative images are registrated to the patient, the surgeon is able to use navigation to plan the surgical pathway from the tip of the instrument to the target site inside the patient. Thus, navigation provides the intuitive correspondence between the patient (physical space), the images (image space that represent the patient) and the tracked surgical instruments. However, when the surgical procedure starts, tissue will change and preoperative data will no longer represent the true patient anatomy. LUS then makes is possible to update the map for guidance and acquire image data that display the true patient anatomy during surgery. Preoperative CT images will, however, still be useful for reference and overview as illustrated in figure 1, showing various display possibilities using LUS and navigation in laparoscopy. An example of simple overlay of tracked surgical tools onto a three-dimensional (3D) volume rendering of computerized tomography (CT) images is shown in figure 1A. In this figure, we used the preoperative 3D CT images for initial in-the-OR planning of the procedure. The view direction of the volume was set by the view direction of the laparoscope. The LUS image could be displayed in the same scene, with an indication of the probe position in yellow. Furthermore, when 3D preoperative images are displayed together with 3D LUS, anatomic shifts can easily be visualized and measured, thereby providing updated information of the true patient anatomy to the surgical team as illustrated in figure 1C. This may improve the accuracy and precision of the procedure. Additionally, the tracked position of the LUS probe can be used to display the corresponding slice from a preoperative CT volume, providing improved overview of the position of the LUS image as shown in figure 1D. Having 3D LUS vailable, it is possible to display these data the same way as traditional orthogonal display of MR and CT volumes, as shown in figure 1E-G. Intraoperative augmented reality visualizations in combination with navigation technology could be valuable for the surgeons (Langø et al., 2008). A possible future development, useful for spotting the true position of lesion and vessels and hence detect anatomic shifts quickly, would be to introduce LUS data into such a multimodal display.

The overall goal of all medical technology mentioned in this chapter is to improve the safety and clinical outcome for the patients. In addition, by introducing technology, it is an aim that the minimal access approach can be feasible for more procedures. Guidance solutions must therefore be designed to improve the work for surgeons and enabling younger/less experienced surgeons to perform surgical procedures with better quality and precision and with increased safety for the patients than achieved without using the technology. We believe that LUS and navigation technology in laparoscopy procedures are such technologies. However, although surgeons believe that LUS has advantages, only 43 % of the respondents in a survey claimed to use it routinely (Våpenstad et al., 2010). The surveyed surgeons were largely positive towards an increased use of LUS in a 5 years perspective and believed that LUS combined with navigation technology would contribute to improving surgical precision of tumor resection.

We present the main technological components involved in navigated ultrasound in laparoscopy. In addition, we provide an overview of ongoing technological research and development related to LUS combined with navigation technology. This chapter could serve as: 1) an introduction for those new to the field of navigated LUS; 2) an overview for those working in the field and; 3) as a reference for those searching for literature on technological developments related to navigation in ultrasound guided laparoscopic surgery.

PubMed[1], Google Scholar[2], and the IEEE database[3] were searched to identify relevant publications from the last ten years. Additional publications were identified by manual

---

[1] www.ncbi.nlm.nih.gov/pubmed/

search through the references from the key papers found. In this chapter we focus on publications published in the last five years. The search was limited to navigated LUS including variations such as ultrasonography, sonography, and echography, in combination with key words such as navigation, tracking, endoscopy, and 3D ultrasound. Publications covering only 3D ultrasound acquisition (e.g. volume estimations and visualization) were not included. Furthermore, we excluded papers on percutaneous techniques, open surgery approach, transrectal ultrasound guided laparoscopic prostatectomy, and transcutaneous guided radiofrequency ablation procedures. Furthermore, when groups have published same studies in both scientific papers and conference presentations, we only included data from the full peer reviewed paper in the overview.

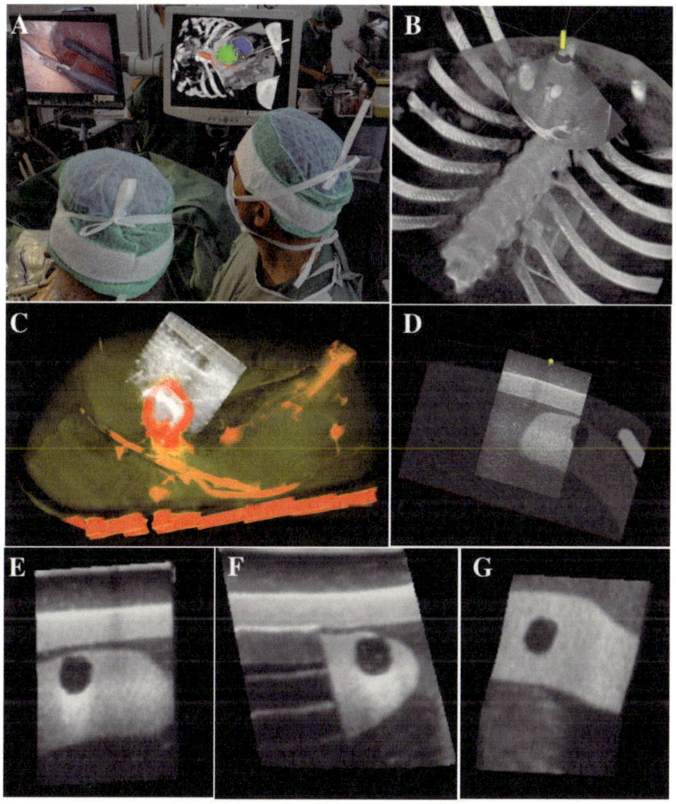

Fig. 1. Illustration of visualization methods for navigation in laparoscopy. A) Navigation during adrenalectomy using preoperative CT (3D and 2D). B) Live animal model (pig) experiment showing navigated LUS combined with preoperative images (CT volume rendering). This solves the orientation problems and improves overview . C) Multimodal display of 3D LUS (volume rendering) and 3D CT from an *ex vivo* experiment showing that the tumor position has changed. D) Anyplane slicing from CT controlled by the LUS probe and overlaying the LUS onto the corresponding CT slice (phantom). E-G) Orthogonal slices from a 3D LUS scan (phantom).

[2] scholar.google.com

[3] ieeexplore.ieee.org

2. Navigated ultrasound in laparoscopic surgery

We introduce all the relevant technologies related to navigated LUS and present a literature overview.

2.1 LUS probes

Intraoperative ultrasound systems are inexpensive, compact, mobile, and have no requirements for special facilities in the operating room (OR) compared to MRI or CT. Ultrasound image quality is continuously improving and for certain cases (e.g. liver) LUS could obtain image quality comparable to what is achieved in neurosurgery, as the probe is placed directly on the surface of the organ. In neurosurgery, the image quality of ultrasound has been demonstrated previously by our group (Unsgaard et al., 2002). The most common LUS probe is a flexible 2- or 4-way array, linear or curved, with a frequency range of 5-10 MHz. Typical imaging depths are in the range 0-10 cm, but with 5MHz deeper imaging can be performed. The LUS transducers usually have a footprint of less than 10 mm wide to fit through trocars and 20-50 mm long. They can be manipulated at the shaft allowing real time images at user-controlled orientations and positions, depending only on the specific probe configuration. Figure 2 shows various configurations of LUS probes, while Table 1 provides an overview of currently available probes.

Most LUS probes can be sterilized (Rutala, 1996) either with Sterrad, ethylene oxide, 2% glutaraldehyde, or Cidex OPA (Benzenedicarboxaldehyde, Ethicon Inc., USA). As an alternative, they can be put into sterile sheaths. Some probes also support low-temperature hydrogen peroxide gas plasma sterilization techniques. Gas plasma sterilization is shorter, and aeration and ventilation of the probe after sterilization is not necessary.

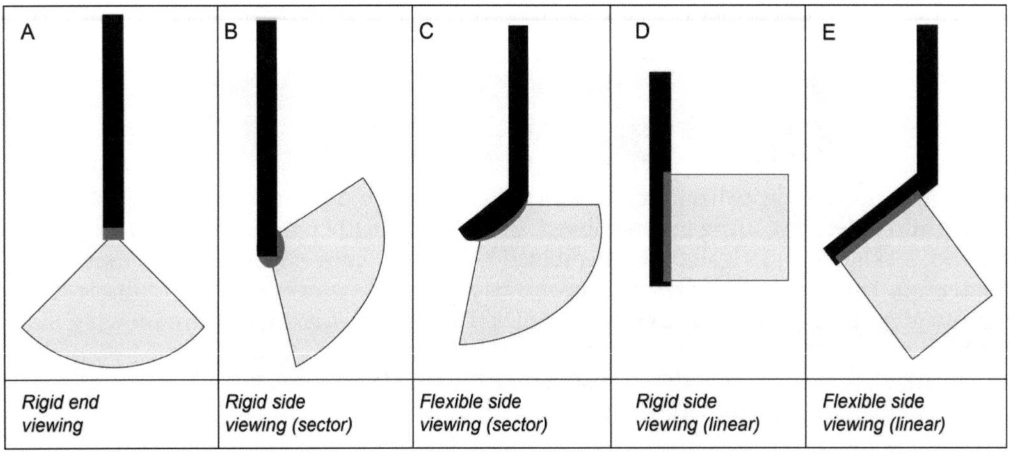

Fig. 2. Configurations of different LUS probes (Solberg et al., 2009). Option B can also be forward viewing like the Toshiba probe in Table 1.

Vendor	Probe	Frequency	Type of probe (see Fig. 2)	Transducer length, scan angle, other
Aloka	UST-52109	3-7.5 MHz	A	10 mm, 90°
	UST-5524-LAP	4-10 MHz	E	38 mm
	UST-5526L-7.5	5-10 MHz	D	33 mm
	UST-5536-7.5	5-10 MHz	E	38 mm
BK Medical	8666-RF	5-10 MHz	E	30 mm, Puncture and biopsy guide
Hitachi	EUP OL531	5-10 MHz	C	120°, Biopsy and therapy
Toshiba	PEF 704LA	5, 7.5, 10 MHz	E	34 mm
	PVM 787LA	5, 7.5, 10 MHz	B	85°
Gore	Tetrad VersaPlane	7.5 MHz (center frequency)	E	56 mm
Philips / ATL	LAP L9-5	5-9 MHz	E	NA
Esaote	LP323	4-13 MHz	E	NA

Table 1. LUS probe models from various manufacturers. Relevant specifications are also given.

2.2 Limitations with 2D LUS technology

Challenges with conventional (2D) LUS include the limited field of view compared to CT or MRI, and that LUS is dependent on the surgeons' experience and competence level in both performing the examination and interpreting the images. A limited field of view contributes to interpretation difficulties, especially for surgeons not experienced with ultrasound. An important factor is the difficulty in interpreting the orientation of the LUS image in relation to other images such as the video laparoscope and preoperative images.

Ultrasound, compared to CT and MRI, usually has a lower signal-to-noise ratio, and the specular nature of ultrasound images may cause shadowing, multiple reflection artifacts, and variable contrast. The introduction of ultrasound contrast agents and new processing techniques like ultrasound based elastography processing (strain) could provide new possibilities due to further improved image quality and structure detection.

The LUS probe is inserted through a trocar and the transducer shaft can only be manipulated along that pivot point where the proximal shaft is fixed at the insertion port. When the probe is pivoted the plane of view is changed and this can cause disorientation. Thus, constant reference to the orientation of the probe on the laparoscopic image and/or some other reference are necessary. The limited access to the organs from different angles due to trocar placement often makes it difficult to obtain a complete overview of the organ using conventional 2D LUS. One of the limitations with 2D LUS is difficulty in maintaining a view of the distal part of an instrument. This problem could be solved by real time 3D LUS (next section) or navigation combined with 2D LUS as will be presented later.

2.3 3D LUS

Real-time monitoring of the position of surgical instruments in relation to the patient's current anatomy is necessary for accurate image guided therapy. This could be achieved using 3D LUS. There are different methods to obtain 3D LUS. One method would be to make use of 3D LUS probes, which are not yet available commercially. But papers about development of such probes have been published (Light et al., 2005). 3D LUS can also be obtained by freehand scanning over the area of interest and tracking the LUS image as mentioned previously. The 3D reconstruction process may be implemented in many different ways (Solberg et al., 2007), depending on speed and quality requirements. 3D LUS imaging provides the possibility to slice the volume in any direction (figure 1E-G), providing otherwise physically unobtainable 2D slices. Tracking the LUS probe enables navigation, presented next.

2.4 Navigation

Navigation combines imaging and tracking technology thus enabling steering of surgical tools into the body based on image information and minimal access. Using navigation it is possible to perform visualization of multiple images from different sources as well as instruments in a common scene. To achieve surgical navigation based on preoperative images it is necessary to perform a registration, calibration and tracking. The following sections discuss these procedures.

2.4.1 Registration

Registration is the process of relating images to each other or relating the images to the patient. Using only intraoperative images like ultrasound for navigation purposes, no registration is necessary as the images are acquired within the tracking/patient coordinate system itself (Figure 3). Using preoperative images, registration of the preoperative images to the patient (reference frame attached to the OR table) is required to perform navigated surgery. Such registration is conventionally performed using fiducial markers or anatomical landmarks. The points are marked in both the images and on the patient using a navigation pointer (Figure 3). The registration accuracy, showing the calculated match between preoperative images and the patient is usually provided to the user after the point match is calculated. The error value provides an indication of error when using the preoperative images for guidance. However, this error will increase during surgery due to shifting anatomy. The use of multimodal image display, real time imaging (LUS) in combination with preoperative data, can potentially help detect and correct for possible anatomic shifts. For laparoscopic navigation, LUS vessel data may be used for CT-to-LUS vessel based registration to update the preoperative data for a better fit the patient data (Reinertsen et al., 2007). The reader is referred to the review paper by Maintz and coworkers (Maintz & Viergever, 1998) for further details on registration techniques.

2.4.2 LUS probe calibration

To perform a freehand 3D LUS scan or perform navigated LUS, a calibration procedure must be performed. This procedure determines the location of the LUS image in space in relation to the tracking sensor attached to the LUS probe (Mercier et al., 2005) as shown in

Figure 3. The procedure is crucial for reconstructing an accurate and geometrically correct LUS volume. A precise calibration can be best obtained by scanning a phantom with a known geometry. The features are identified in the ultrasound image of the phantom and these features are also located in physical space. The spatial relationship between the two data sets is computed in the calibration process. Some of the commonly used phantoms for probe calibration are (Mercier et al., 2005):

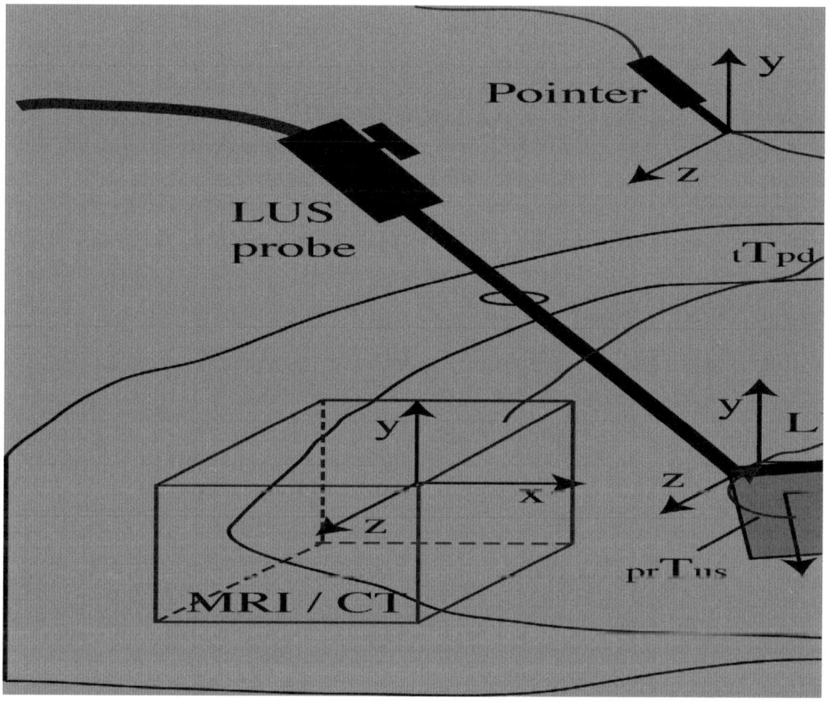

Fig. 3. The various coordinate systems involved to achieve navigated LUS in combination with preoperative data. The transformation matrices (T) shows how the various coordinate systems are linked to the tracking field generator system (arrows). ${}_{t}T_{po}$ is pointer position relative to the tracker, ${}_{t}T_{pd}$ is the preoperative data position after registration to the patient, ${}_{t}T_{pr}$ is the LUS probe position, ${}_{pr}T_{us}$ is the ultrasound image position relative to the LUS probe sensor (the probe calibration procedure establishes this transformation), and ${}_{t}T_{pa}$ is the patient reference sensor position.

- *Single point target and cross wire phantoms*
- *Multiple point targets and cross wire phantoms*
- *2-D shape alignment phantoms*
- *Wall phantoms*

It is possible to bring all the objects in the operating room into a common coordinate system by attaching position sensors to all surgical instruments, including the LUS probe (Figure 3), and a reference position sensor to the patient. However, both registration of preoperative images to the patient and probe calibration affect the overall accuracy of a navigation system (Lindseth et al., 2002; Lindseth et al., 2003). So the registration and calibration procedures must be selected carefully to reduce the error introduced in the navigation system to aid effective and accurate laparoscopic procedures. For a detailed descriptions about the various calibration methods, the reader is referred to Mercier *et al* (Mercier et al., 2005).

2.4.3 Tracking of surgical tools

There are four common technologies for tracking medical instruments: electromagnetic (EM), optical, mechanical arm and acoustic (Cinquin et al., 1995). EM or optical are most commonly used technologies for tracking in medical applications. Optical systems have a high accuracy, but require a free line of sight between the sensors/markers and the cameras. Optical methods are limited to rigid instruments. In laparoscopic surgery, independency from line of sight is important in order to facilitate the tracking of flexible instruments (including LUS probes) inside the human body. For this reason, EM tracking systems are most suitable as they are unaffected by sensor occlusion. However, distortions may occur from metallic objects in the working space that induce perturbations of the EM field. This will be discussed in detail later.

2.4.4 Visualization and display

In general, 3D volumes have a number of display and visualization possibilities that are not dependent upon using navigation technology. Using navigation technology it is, however, possible to steer the display using surgical tools or pointers. In addition, navigation and tracking technology is necessary to track positions of 2D ultrasound probes in order to reconstruct the images into a 3D volume, that can be displayed in various ways. Most medical images relevant in laparoscopy may be displayed either in 2D or 3D (pseudo-3D or true stereoscopic 3D), regardless of the image source being 2D or 3D. In addition, data from several sources/modalities may be displayed together as mentioned. To allow easier presentation of multimodal images, a common method is to extract interesting areas and present these as differently coloured surface models (segmentation).

3D display examples of multimodal images are:

- Rendering of surface models from multiple data sources.
- Volume rendering of one data source, with surface models from other data sources (Figure 1A).
- Volume rendering of multiple data sources (Figure 1C). This usually requires different colouring to distinguish the volumes from each other. Surface models may also be included.

2D display examples of multimodal images:

- One data source in each 2D display. For 3D data sources, each data source may have several 2D displays showing slices in different directions, e.g. axial, coronal and sagittal, as shown in Figure 1E-G.
- Several data sources are shown in each 2D display, the smaller or more detailed sources obscuring others.
- Several data sources in each 2D display using blending with see-through effects (the use of colours is useful).

The physical positions of the data shown in the different 2D views may be linked, and the same position in all views may be marked with a crosshairs or similar. 3D and 2D may also be combined in one 3D display by showing the 2D with correct placement in 3D. Several different 3D volume rendering methods with different rendering speed and quality may be used (Karadayi et al., 2009). Different transfer functions and filters may also improve the volume visualization quality. Fast, relatively high quality volume rendering is available today with graphics processing units (GPUs).

Even with these visualization methods available, the orientation problem in laparoscopy is even more challenging compared to other surgical disciplines. The reason is that the video laparoscope shows an image from a different angle than the LUS probe, neither of them necessarily viewing the patient anatomy at the same angle as the surgeon. Using navigation technology makes it possible to display the LUS data from various directions independently of the ultrasound acquisition direction, which may be important for interpretation of essential structures and lesions (Solberg et al., 2009).

2.5 Literature overview on navigated LUS

Only very few review or overview papers were found that partly covers the topic of navigated LUS, and none of them represent a complete overview on the area. The few relevant reviews were the following:

i. Navigation and computer assisted systems for endoscopic soft tissue surgery (Baumhauer et al., 2008). The paper informs the reader about new trends and technologies in the area of computer-assisted surgery for soft tissues in general. It contains a few references to papers dealing with navigated LUS.
ii. Navigation and image-guided hepatobiliary-pancreatic surgery (Lamadé et al., 2002).
iii. Interventional navigation systems for treatment of unresectable liver tumor (Phee & Yang, 2010). The authors only report one publication on LUS based navigation.

Below we present an overview of findings in the literature, limited to LUS in combination with navigation technology. Included in the overview are study type, tracking method, LUS probe, calibration method of LUS probe, registration method, images / visualization methods, and a brief mention of the main findings from the group.

- Martens (Martens et al., 2010): EM tracking, flexible LUS probe, ex vivo and in vivo studies, automatic multiple cross wire LUS probe calibration, landmark based coarse registration followed by surface registration using ICP. The group is developing a navigation system for laparoscopic liver interventions. They used LUS volume rendering, 3D view of preoperative data and tracked instruments, and 2D LUS image. Main result was a technical system ready for human trials.
- Sindram (Sindram et al., 2010): EM tracking, flexible LUS probe, phantom trainer, no calibration available, and no registration presented. They tried to determine whether using a magnetic tracking system improves accuracy during needle placement. They used stereoscopic 3D display and needle trajectory visualization. They reported perfect targeting of 5 mm lesions by novice surgeons.
- Solberg (Solberg et al., 2009): EM tracking, flexible LUS probe, phantom studies, 2D shape alignment calibration, and fiducial based registration (CT-model). The group is develpoing a navigated LUS system and assessed the accuracy of 3D LUS and EM tracking accuracy in a realistic OR setting. They demonstrated slicing, anyplane,

multivolume, volume rendering, and surface view visualization. They found the 3D LUS accurate in a phantom set-up, 1.6% to 3.6% volume deviation from the phantom specifications and little disturbance to EM field.

- Feuerstein (Feuerstein et al., 2009): EM and optical tracking, flexible LUS probe, system description, single wall calibration (Prager et al., 1998), and no registration described. They reported mainly on a method for correction of intraoperative magnetic distortion that can be applied to improve LUS based navigation. The overall goal was a 3D LUS system for augmented reality in laparoscopic surgery. No visualization method were described or demonstrated. They found that modeling the poses of the transducer tip in relation to the transducer shaft allowed them to reliably detect and significantly reduce EM tracking errors.
- Langø (Langø et al., 2008): EM tracking, flexible LUS probe, system description, 2D shape alignment calibration, and fiducial based registration (CT, patient). The publication was mainly a technical development (hardware and software) description of a navigation system for laparoscopy, including LUS component. They showed slicing, anyplane, multivolume, volume rendering, and surface view visualizations. The authors presented clinical feasibility from pilot trials.
- Hildebrand (Hildebrand et al., 2008): EM tracking, flexible LUS probe, ex vivo studies, and manual landmark registration (CT to physical space of porcine model setup). The group was developing a navigation system for laparoscopic liver therapy with focus on radio frequency ablation. They demonstrated 3D surface view of planning data, overlay of navigated needle and 2D LUS on 3D surface view of planning data. They found that advanced laparoscopic ultrasound skills are the basis for accurate RFA probe placement.
- Nakamoto, Nakada, Sato (Nakada et al., 2003; Nakamoto et al., 2008; Sato et al., 2001): EM tracking, in vitro and in vivo studies, 2D shape alignment calibration, and no registration method mentioned. The group showed 3D LUS based augmented reality visualization during laparoscopic surgery and demonstrated a calibration method for intraoperative magnetic distortion that can be applied during LUS acquisitions. LUS volume rendering was used as a visualization approach. They found that data acquisition time shortened with improved distortion correction. Their proposed method corrects magnetic distortion with an accuracy of 3 mm or less within 2 minutes.
- Konishi (Konishi et al., 2007): EM and optical tracking, flexible LUS probe, in vivo studies, 2D shape alignment calibration, and landmark based registration (CT-endoscopic views). They evaluated the usefulness and accuracy of a navigation system in an animal model. 3D LUS was overlaid on endoscopic view (augmented reality visualization) and vessel structures were displayed on preoperative CT data. They reported that the rapid calibration method was effective and it corrects magnetic distortion with accuracy of 2 mm.
- Hildebrand (Hildebrand et al., 2007): EM tracking, flexible LUS probe, ex vivo studies, no probe calibration available, and no registration method were mentioned. They evaluated an EM navigation system for laparoscopic interventions using a perfusable ex vivo artificial tumor model. Overlay of tracked instrument on 2D LUS image were performed. They concluded that laparoscopic ultrasound guided navigation is technically feasible.
- Estepar (Estépar et al., 2007; Estépar et al., 2007): EM tracking, in vivo studies, single wall calibration, and fiducial based registration (CT-LUS). Ultrasound based navigation system

for transgastric access procedures were described in the publication. Visualization was performed with 3D surface model from CT with tracked probe overlaid on the model. They were able to report successful navigation for transgastric access.

- Bao (Bao et al., 2004): Optical tracking, rigid side looker LUS probe, phantom studies, plane mapping calibration, and no registration method described. The group was developing a laparoscopic radiofrequency ablation guidance system. They demonstrated 3D LUS volume rendering and overlay of tracked instrument on 2D and 3D LUS image. Targeting accuracy was reported to be 5-10 mm (size of error in missing targets).
- Kleeman, Birth (Birth et al., 2004; Kleemann et al., 2006): EM tracking, in vivo studies, no probe calibration available, and no registration mentioned. The authors wanted to transfer navigated parenchyma dissection from open surgery to the laparoscopic technique. They utilized navigation line overlaid on the 2D LUS with a function to indicate out of plane dissection. They showed that this was feasible for achieving increased precision in laparoscopic liver dissection.
- Leven (Leven et al., 2005): EM tracking, rigid LUS probe, ex vivo studies, single wall calibration, and no registration described. Their goal was to develop a versatile telerobotic surgical system useful for multiple procedures. They used 2D LUS viewed as a picture-in-picture insert or as an overlay on endoscopic video. 3D LUS overlay on endoscopic video was also implemented. They found that experienced surgeons performed better with freehand ultrasound. Experienced and novice surgeons performed similarly with robotic assistance and robotic assistance required longer time for surgeons to identify lesions.
- Krucker (Krucker et al., 2005): EM tracking, flexible LUS probe, phantom studies, single point cross wire calibration, and fiducial based registration (CT to LUS). They used EM tracking to register LUS to preoperative CT. They performed overlay of LUS with preoperative CT and the registrations could be visualized together with tracked instruments. Fast and accurate registration was obtained using a tracked laparoscope with EM tracking.
- Bao (Bao et al., 2005): Optical tracking, rigid side looker LUS probe, phantom studies, plane mapping calibration (Bao et al., 2004), and fiducial based registration (CT to LUS) was used. The authors attempted to perform registration of ultrasound to CT for image-guided laparoscopic liver procedures. They used various CT renderings and visualization of 2D LUS placed in 3D CT. They found an average localization error of 5.3 mm.
- Ellsmere (Ellsmere et al., 2003; Ellsmere et al., 2004): EM tracking, flexible LUS probe, in vivo studies, single point cross wire calibration, and anatomical landmark based registration (CT to LUS). They demonstrated on the development fo a system for orienting and visualizing LUS images better. They used ultrasound 2D images and volume rendering visualization with respect to CT angiograms. They concluded that visual orientation information to the surgeon significantly improved the ability to interpret LUS images.
- Wilheim (Wilheim et al., 2003): EM tracking, flexible LUS probe, in vitro and in vivo studies, no calibration or registration method were mentioned. The authors presented an evaluation of an EM navigated LUS and a comparison of 3D navigated transcutaneous ultrasound and 3D CT. They used LUS volume rendering visualization. They found that navigated LUS was superior to both transcutaneous 3D ultrasound and 2D LUS.

- Harms (Harms et al., 2001): EM tracking, linear flexible LUS probe, ex vivo and in vivo studies, no calibration or registration method were mentioned. The group performed 3D ultrasound of liver lesions, comparing 3D LUS to 3D CT. They used 2D slicing and LUS volume rendering visualization. They found that LUS slightly underestimated the volume of the region of interest and that LUS was more accurate than transcutaneous ultrasound.

In summary, these publications show that navigated LUS has several advantages in laparoscopic guidance compared to conventional 2D LUS, especially due to the orientation challenges. The further advancement of soft tissue navigation requires surgeons, engineers, and perhaps radiologists, to collaborate more closely, inside and outside the OR. Specific surgical procedures have to be identified, where current technological possibilities will fulfill user demands as a tool for obtaining improved patient care. From the literature it seems that authors have targeted laparoscopic liver therapy guidance as one of the most important applications, where the demands for navigated LUS is emphasized. There is a general lack of assessment protocols that can be used to evaluate the technological solutions to show a potential clinical benefit to the patient and/or the surgical staff. This is of course connected to the fact that most publications are in early development phases. Nevertheless, such clinical study protocols should be developed early during research to enable possibilities for proper clinical assessment of navigated LUS.

2.6 Image fusion

3D ultrasound integrated with preoperative images can help interpreting the content of the LUS images, as well as the position, in correspondence with surrounding anatomy. We have previously mentioned that image fusion techniques can make it easier to perceive the integration of two or more volumes in the same display (monitor), compared to mentally fusing the two volumes that are displayed on separate monitors (Solberg et al., 2009). Ideally, relevant information should not only include anatomical structures for reference and pathological structures to be targeted (CT/MRI and ultrasound tissue), but also important structures to be avoided, like blood vessels (depicted with CT/MR contrast, ultrasound Doppler). We believe that such features will be important when visualizing LUS data together with preoperative CT data from a patient during surgery. The ultrasound data will show updated information that the surgeon relies on during surgery, while advantages from preoperative data, such as better overview and understanding of the anatomy and pathology, are also considered. Nevertheless, this type of multivolume visualization demands fast rendering algorithms, e.g. using GPU. Such methods are becoming more available as GPU application interfaces are being developed and tested on various brands of GPU and computer system platforms. Multimodal imaging may be achieved with 2D slices or 3D surface models also, requiring less processing power than multivolume 3D renderings.

2.7 Virtual endoscopy

A technique that could have potential in laparoscopy is "virtual endoscopy" (Shahidi et al., 2002) or image-enhanced endoscopy. This approach uses computer graphics to render the view seen by a navigated video laparoscope inside the abdomen, based on a representation of the cavity calculated from preoperative MRI or CT images. Using segmented structures (e.g. tumor and vessels) overlaid the real laparoscopic video is often termed augmented reality or multimodal image fusion visualization (Konishi et al., 2007; Scheuering et al., 2003). Such a view may help the surgeons to quickly interpret important information beyond the surface of the organs as seen by the conventional video camera. More research into segmentation of anatomic and pathologic structures may improve the usefulness of e.g. overlay or side-by-side view of virtual endoscopy and tracked laparoscopic images. Combining this with LUS could help detect organ shifts and also augment the scene view further for the surgeon, providing more details in depth and in real time.

To make it easier to understand what is beyond the surface of organs as seen in the laparoscope during surgery, navigation and image fusion can be used as shown in figure 4. Segmented structures from 3D CT can be gradually overlaid the video laparoscopic image, showing important information about lesion and vessel position inside the organ. This may improve the surgical approach both due to optimal resection and the avoidance of bleedings.

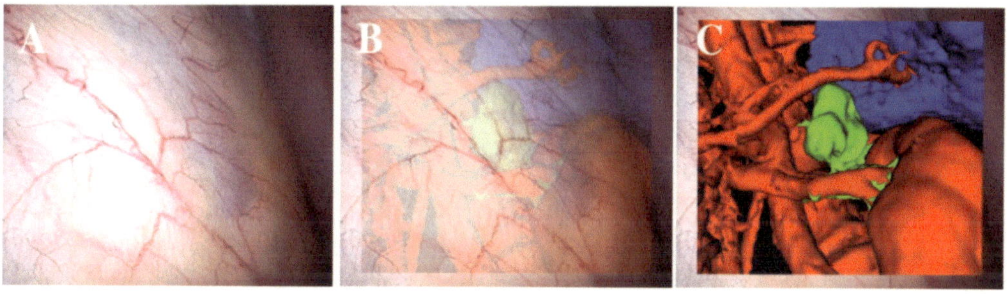

Fig. 4. Augmented reality example showing segmented structures from a CT volume overlaid the video laparoscope image, making it possible to see beyond the surface of the organ. This makes it possible to perform optimal resection planning during a laparoscopic adrenalectomy.

2.8 Challenges - Organ shifts and tissue deformations

The main challenges of navigated surgery of soft tissues are shifts due to manipulation and gravity. Movement of anatomy such as that caused by blood flow pulsation, breathing and induction of pneumoepritoneum in laparoscopy could mean that the preoperative images no longer match the intraoperative target anatomy of the patient. We have found that pneumoperitoneum causes a shift of the liver in an animal model (pig) of up to approximately 3 cm (no significant deformation, unpublished data). Pulsation and breathing causes smaller but repetitive displacements in anatomy. Important approaches in order to solve the problem of displaced anatomy due to surgical manipulations, probably the largest shifts, are navigation technology combined with LUS. Intraoperative ultrasound is becoming routine in some surgical disciplines, e.g. neurosurgery (Unsgaard et al., 2006). Another approach is to update or morph preoperative data based on intraoperative ultrasound (Bucholz et al., 1997; Reinertsen et al., 2007) to better match the intraoperative situation. This is a computationally expensive method, and also prone to errors difficult to detect, i.e. changes to parts of the volume cannot be easily verified during the procedure. Shifts detected by LUS could for instance be utilized to colour code preoperative data voxels to make the surgeon aware of deformations and shifts.

In laparoscopy, we have experienced that when the lesion is located in the retroperitoneum, only minor shifts in anatomy are detected (Mårvik et al., 2004), which may be compensated by using 3D ultrasound to acquire updated maps of the anatomy. Nevertheless, tissue motion and deformations during surgery require continuous correction and update of images for constant and reliable navigation accuracy. Freehand 3D ultrasound systems can be extended to 4D ultrasound images and these 4D ultrasound images can be used to determine the liver motion and deformation caused by respiration by using a non-rigid registration method (Nakamoto et al., 2007).

Application of soft tissue modeling methods is becoming a promising manner to enable continuous motion compensation during navigated surgery (Carter et al., 2005; Hawkes et al., 2005). Mathematical models are able to describe tissue behavior to a certain degree of accuracy during a procedure based on various parameters estimated for the organ. Rigid based deformation techniques can only describe global changes, while spline-based approaches can also capture local variances of tissue deformation by varying the position of a few control points (landmarks). Such methods are also used in virtual simulators for training laparoscopic skills (Kühnapfel et al., 2000). 4D models that use gating techniques or tracking technology to track the patients' breathing and/or blood pulsation enable image-guided therapy with higher accuracy and security.

2.9 Challenges - EM tracking accuracy

One of the major challenges with EM tracking is that it is vulnerable to disturbances from ferromagnetic interference sources in the surroundings, which may influence the accuracy of the system. Several groups have performed static and dynamic accuracy evaluations of different EM and optical trackers (Frantz et al., 2003; Nafis et al., 2006; Nafis et al., 2008; Schmerber & Chassat, 2001), which provide useful data for accuracy comparisons. EM trackers in the OR are subjected to distortion from several sources, and the impact of the level of interference may vary between the different trackers. A number of papers deal with distortions to the EM tracking systems from metals (Hummel et al., 2005; Kirsch et al., 2006; Nafis et al., 2006), surgical instruments (Hummel et al., 2002; Schicho et al., 2005), ultrasound probes (Hastenteufel et al., 2006; Hummel et al., 2002; Schicho et al., 2005), OR tables (Hummel et al., 2005; Nafis et al., 2008) and OR environments (Wilson et al., 2007). In summary, these papers also show that the EM trackers robustness regarding distortion sources have improved significantly over the latest years. Using EM tracking in a conventional OR equipped for laparoscopy, distortions would normally be in the milimeter range, while in ORs with special equipment like a C-arm inside the surgical field, distoritons may be in the centimeter range (Wilson et al., 2007) (and own unpublished data).

One group (Hastenteufel et al., 2006) showed that 2D ultrasound probes does not affect EM tracking system accuracy significantly compared to the more complex 3D ultrasound probes when using the Flock of Birds® (Ascension Technology, USA) tracking system. However, they found that the 2D probes significantly affected the Aurora® (NDI, Canada) tracking system accuracy. This is most likely due to the fact that Aurora is based on alternating current technology and Flock of Birds uses pulsed direct current technology, so they will have different advantages and drawbacks when used in various environments. Schicho *et al* (Schicho et al., 2005) also showed that a 2D ultrasound probe affects EM tracking accuracy in an ideal setup where the ultrasound probe is the only distortion factor. We have shown previously that the error introduced by a LUS probe does not add significantly to the error of the Aurora tracking system, compared to the contribution from the OR table and surrounding error sources in an intraoperative experimental setup (Solberg et al., 2009). The largest distortion factor in our OR setup was most likely the OR table, being quite close to the Aurora field generator and sensor. Although equipment in the OR may affect EM positioning accuracy, this challenge can be reduced and the overall benefit of navigated 3D ultrasound using EM tracking seems sufficient to be further explored in laparoscopy.

It is therefore important to assess the accuracy, not only for each system, but also for each new location where the system is to be used. If there are disturbances that are constant and may be properly characterized, they may be compensated using static correction schemes (Chung et al., 2004; Kindratenko, 2000). These correction schemes require a set of distributed measurements within the tracking volume and corresponding reference measurements to compute a distortion function.

Since the interference depends on the surroundings, it must be characterized for each new location and the correction scheme must be adapted accordingly. In addition, if the environment changes during the procedure, e.g. by introduction of additional equipment, this must be taken into account. One of the earlier attempts to compensating dynamic errors intraoperatively involved focusing on the region of interest alone to apply the distortion model (Konishi et al., 2007; Nakamoto et al., 2008). A more recent approach to detect and reduce dynamic EM tracking errors intraoperatively makes use of a tracking redundancy and a model based approach instead of a pre-computed distortion function (Feuerstein et al., 2009).

2.10 Other error sources

In addition to tracking errors, probe calibration is an important error source in ultrasound based image guided surgery. Incorrect probe calibration implies that an image point will be displaced from its "true" position in the navigation system display. If the probe is shifted/rotated, the same shift/rotation occurs to the displacement. Probe calibration may be related to various error sources (Mercier et al., 2005) and is perhaps the largest source of error in 3D freehand ultrasound acquisitions (Lindseth et al., 2002). Additional sources of error in navigated LUS are:

- Sensor attachment repeatability. EM trackers are usually integrated into the probe so that this is not an important factor if they are made in such a way that a unique adapter is fitted to each probe.
- Reference frame attachment to the patient and/or OR table. The OR team may easily bump into this equipment, displacing it relative to the patient.
- Synchronization in time between position data and ultrasound images during acquisition (3D freehand scanning) and navigation.
- Sound speed variations in tissue, which is less important in relatively homogenous soft tissues. This parameter is especially important when reconstructing freehand tracked 2D ultrasound slices into a 3D volume.
- Thickness of the ultrasound plane, which could lower the quality of the 3D volume and cause less accurate determination of structure positions, especially at large depths in the images.

The delicacy, precision, and extent of the work the surgeon can perform based on image information, rely on his/her confidence in the overall clinical accuracy and the anatomical or pathological visualization. The overall clinical accuracy in image-guided surgery is the difference between where a surgical tool is located (orientation and position) relative to a structure as indicated in the images presented to the surgeon, and where the tool is actually located relative to the same structure inside the patient. This overall accuracy is difficult to assess in a clinical setting, due to the lack of fixed and well-defined landmarks inside the patient that can be reached accurately by a tracked instrument. One solution is to estimate the system's overall accuracy in a controlled laboratory setting using precisely built phantoms. In order to conclude on the potential clinical accuracy, the differences between the clinical and the laboratory settings must be carefully examined (Lindseth et al., 2002). It is crucial that the user of image based navigation systems is aware of the potential error sources and limitations in accuracy, e.g. expected accuracy and maximum differences in real position of instrument tip versus position displayed by the navigation system.

3. Summary

Being a relatively new area of research, it is interesting to note that the number of active research groups in this field seems to be 10-11. Based on the overview, we have been able to identify the key issues and also spot the future possibilities in the area to help improve the surgical scenario in the OR. Based on our literature findings and almost two decades working with surgeons on developments for advanced laparoscopic surgery, a complete system designed for navigated LUS could be used according to the following clinical scenario:

- The preoperative data is imported and reconstructed into 3D; several structures and organs are segmented automatically (e.g. vessels from contrast CT scan) or semi-automatically (e.g. seed point set inside the tumor).
- A quick plan is made from the visualization in the navigation system just prior to surgery, perhaps in the OR during other preparations.
- Registration is performed without fiducials using a pointer (orientation of patient) and two landmarks for a rough first approximation.
- Before mobilizing the target organ (e.g. the liver) a 3D LUS scan of major vessels near or around the tumor is performed.
- The LUS images are reconstructed into 3D and an automatic vessel based registration (CT-to-ultrasound) is performed to fine tune the registration.
- Augmented reality visualization, e.g. on/off overlay of preoperative data and LUS on the video laparoscope view is preformed as needed by the surgeons during the procedure
- 3D LUS scans are updated a few times during the procedure, while the real time 2D LUS image is available as either:
    - A full size image with a corresponding indication in a 3D CT rendering of its orientation and position, or
    - An overlay on the video laparoscope view with or without elements from the CT data (segmented structures for instance).

For rigid organ navigation, a single preoperative scan, highly accurate tracking (optical), and rigid surgical tools are sufficient to guide the procedure. However, for soft tissue navigation, additional tools are needed due to deformation and mobile organs in the abdominal cavity, resulting in more complex systems and additional devices in the OR. LUS can provide real time behind-the-surface information (tissue, blood flow, elasticity). When combined with advanced visualization techniques and preoperative images, LUS can enhance an augmented reality scene to include updated images of details, important for high precision surgery thus enhancing the perception for surgeons during minimal access therapy. LUS integrated with miniaturized tracking technology is likely to play an important role in guiding future laparoscopic surgery.

4. Acknowledgments

This work was supported by SINTEF, the Ministry of Health and Social Affairs of Norway through the National Centre of 3D Ultrasound in Surgery (Trondheim, Norway) and the project 196726/V50 *eMIT* (*enhanced Minimally Invasive Therapy*) in the FRIMED program of the Research Council of Norway.

5. References

Bao P, Warmath J, Galloway R, Jr., & Herline A. (2005). Ultrasound-to-computer-tomography registration for image-guided laparoscopic liver surgery. *Surg Endosc*, Vol. 19, No. 3, pp. 424-9.

Bao P, Warmath JR, Poulose B, Galloway J, Robert L, & Herline AJ. (2004). Tracked ultrasound for laparoscopic surgery. *Proceedings SPIE Medical Imaging 2004: Visualization, Image-Guided Procedures, and Display*, Vol. 5367, No. 1, pp. 237- 46.

Baumhauer M, Feuerstein M, Meinzer HP, & Rassweiler J. (2008). Navigation in Endoscopic Soft Tissue Surgery: Perspectives and Limitations. *Journal of Endourology*, Vol. 22, No. 4, pp. 751-66.

Birth M, Kleemann M, Hildebrand P, & Bruch HP. (2004). Intraoperative online navigation of dissection of the hepatical tissue—a new dimension in liver surgery? *Proceedings of Computer Assisted Radiology and Surgery (CARS)*, Vol. 1268, No. 2004, pp. 770-74.

Bucholz RD, Yeh DD, Trobaugh J, McDurmott LL, Sturm CD, Baumann C, Henderson JM, Levy A, & Kessman P. (1997). The correction of stereotactic inaccuracy caused by brain shift using an intraoperative ultrasound device. *Lecture Notes in Computer Science (MICCAI)*, Vol. 1205, No. 1997, pp. 459-66.

Carter TJ, Sermesant M, Cash DM, Barratt DC, Tanner C, & Hawkes DJ. (2005). Application of soft tissue modelling to image-guided surgery. *Med Eng Phys*, Vol. 27, No., pp. 893-909.

Chung AJ, Edwards PJ, Deligianni F, & Yang GZ. (2004). Freehand cocalibration of optical and electromagnetic trackers for navigated bronchoscopy. *Medical Imaging and Augmented Reality, Proceedings*, Vol. 3150, No., pp. 320-28.

Cinquin P, Bainville E, Barbe C, Bittar E, Bouchard V, Bricault L, Champleboux G, Chenin M, Chevalier L, Delnondedieu Y, Desbat L, Dessenne V, Hamadeh A, Henry D, Laieb N, Lavallee S, Lefebvre JM, Leitner F, Menguy Y, Padieu F, Peria O, Poyet A, Promayon M, Rouault S, Sautot P, Troccaz J, & Vassal P. (1995). Computer assisted medical interventions. *IEEE Eng Med Biol Magazine*, Vol. 14, No., pp. 254–63.

Ellsmere J, Stoll J, Rattner D, Brooks D, Kane R, Wells W, Kikinis R, & Vosburgh KG. A Navigation System for Augmenting Laparoscopic Ultrasound. Int Conf Med Image Comput Comput Assist Interv (MICCAI), 2003. pp. 184-91.

Ellsmere J, Stoll J, Wells W, 3rd, Kikinis R, Vosburgh K, Kane R, Brooks D, & Rattner D. (2004). A new visualization technique for laparoscopic ultrasonography. *Surgery*, Vol. 136, No. 1, pp. 84-92.

Estépar RSJ, Stylopoulos N, Ellis RE, Samset E, Westin CF, Thompson C, & Vosburgh K. (2007). Towards scarless surgery: An endoscopic ultrasound navigation system for transgastric access procedures. *Computer Aided Surgery*, Vol. 12, No. 6, pp. 311 - 24.

Estépar RSJ, Stylopoulos N, Ellis RE, Samset E, Westin CF, Thompson C, & Vosburgh K. (2007). Towards Scarless Surgery: An Endoscopic-Ultrasound Navigation System for Transgastric Access Procedures. *Lecture Notes in Computer Science (MICCAI)*, Vol. 4190, No., pp. 445–53.

Feuerstein M, Reichl T, Vogel J, Traub J, & Navab N. (2009). Magneto-Optical Tracking of Flexible Laparoscopic Ultrasound: Model-Based Online Detection and Correction of Magnetic Tracking Errors. *IEEE Trans Med Imaging*, Vol. 28, No. 6, pp. 951-67.

Frantz DD, Wiles AD, Leis SE, & Kirsch SR. (2003). Accuracy assessment protocols for electromagnetic tracking systems. *Phys Med Biol*, Vol. 48, No. 14, pp. 2241–51.

Harms J, Feussner H, Baumgartner M, Schneider A, Donhauser M, & Wessels G. (2001). Three-dimensional navigated laparoscopic ultrasonography. *Surg Endosc*, Vol. 15, No. 12, pp. 1459–62.

Hastenteufel M, Vetter M, Meinzer HP, & Wolf I. (2006). Effect of 3d ultrasound probes on the accuracy of electromagnetic tracking systems. *Ultrasound Med Biol*, Vol. 32, No., pp. 1359-68.

Hawkes DJ, Barratt D, Blackall JM, Chan C, Edwards PJ, Rhode K, Penney GP, McClelland J, & Hill DLG. (2005). Tissue deformation and shape models in image-guided interventions: a discussion paper. *Medical Image Analysis*, Vol. 9, No., pp. 163-75.

Hildebrand P, Martens V, Schweikard A, Schlichting S, Besirevic A, Kleemann M, Roblick U, Mirow L, Burk C, & Bruch HP. (2007). Evaluation of an online navigation system for laparoscopic interventions in a perfused ex vivo artificial tumor model of the liver. *HPB (Oxford)*, Vol. 9, No. 3, pp. 190-4.

Hildebrand P, Schlichting S, Martens V, Besirevic A, Kleemann M, Roblick U, Mirow L, Burk C, Schweikard A, & Bruch HP. (2008). Prototype of an intraoperative navigation and documentation system for laparoscopic radiofrequency ablation: first experiences. *Eur J Surg Oncol*, Vol. 34, No. 4, pp. 418-21.

Hummel J, Figl M, Kollmann C, Bergmann H, & Birkfellner W. (2002). Evaluation of a miniature electromagnetic position tracker. *Med Phys*, Vol. 29, No. 10, pp. 2205-12.

Hummel JB, Bax MR, Figl ML, Kang Y, Maurer CJ, Birkfellner WW, Bergmann H, & Shahidi R. (2005). Design and application of an assessment protocol for electromagnetic tracking systems. *Phys Med Biol*, Vol. 32, No. 7, pp. 2371–9.

Jakimowicz JJ. (2006). Intraoperative ultrasonography in open and laparoscopic abdominal surgery: an overview. *Surg Endosc*, Vol. 20 Suppl 2, No., pp. S425-35.

Jakimowicz JJ, & Ruers TJM. (1991). Ultrasound-Assisted Laparoscopic Cholecystectomy: Preliminary Experience. *Dig Surg*, Vol. 8, No., pp. 114-17.

Karadayi K, Managuli R, & Kim Y. (2009). Three-Dimensional Ultrasound From Acquisition to Visualization and From Algorithms to Systems. *Biomedical Engineering, IEEE Reviews*, Vol. 2, No., pp. 23-39.

Kindratenko V. (2000). A survey of electromagnetic position tracker calibration techniques. *Virtual Reality*, Vol. 5, No. 3, pp. 169-82.

Kirsch SR, Schilling C, & Brunner G. Assesment of metallic distortions of an electromagnetic tracking system. In SPIE (Society of Photo-Optical Instrumentation Engineers) Proceedings, 2006. p. 61410J.

Kleemann M, Hildebrand P, Birth M, & Bruch HP. (2006). Laparoscopic ultrasound navigation in liver surgery: technical aspects and accuracy. *Surg Endosc*, Vol. 20, No. 5, pp. 726-9.

Konishi K, Nakamoto M, Kakeji Y, Tanoue K, Kawanaka H, Yamaguchi S, Ieiri S, Sato Y, Maehara Y, Tamura S, & Hashizume M. (2007). A real-time navigation system for laparoscopic surgery based on three-dimensional ultrasound using magneto-optic hybrid tracking configuration. *IJCARS*, Vol. 2, No. 1, pp. 1-10.

Krucker J, Viswanathan A, Borgert J, Glossop N, Yang Y, & Wood BJ. (2005). An electro-magnetically tracked laparoscopic ultrasound for multi modality minimally invasive surgery. *Proceedings of Computer Assisted Radiology and Surgery (CARS)*, Vol. 1281, No. 2005, pp. 746-51.

Kühnapfel U, Çakmak HK, & Maaß H. (2000). Endoscopic surgery training using virtual reality and deformable tissue simulation. *Computer & Graphics*, Vol. 24, No., pp. 671-82.

Lamadé W, Vetter M, Hassenpflug P, Thorn M, Meinzer H-P, & Herfarth C. (2002). Navigation and image-guided HBP surgery: a review and preview. *J Hepatobiliary Pancreat Surg*, Vol. 9, No., pp. 592–99.

Langø T, Tangen GA, Mårvik R, Ystgaard B, Yavuz Y, Kaspersen JH, Solberg OV, & Hernes TAN. (2008). Navigation in laparoscopy - prototype research platform for improved image-guided surgery. *Minimally Invasive Therapy and Allied Technologies (MITAT)*, Vol. 17, No. 1, pp. 17-33.

Leven J, Burschka D, Kumar R, Zhang G, Blumenkranz S, Dai XD, Awad M, Hager GD, Marohn M, Choti M, Hasser CJ, & Taylor RH. (2005). Davinci canvas: A telerobotic surgical system with integrated, robot-assisted, laparoscopic ultrasound capability. *Lecture Notes in Computer Science (MICCAI)*, Vol. 3749, No., pp. 811-18.

Light ED, Idriss SF, Sullivan KF, Wolf PD, & Smith1 SW. (2005). Real-time 3D laparoscopic ultrasonography. *Ultrason Imaging*, Vol. 27 No., pp. 129–44.

Lindseth F, Langø T, Bang J, & Hernes TAN. (2002). Accuracy evaluation of a 3D ultrasound-based neuronavigation system. *Comp Aided Surg*, Vol. 7, No. 4, pp. 197-200.

Lindseth F, Tangen G, Langø T, & Bang J. (2003). Probe calibration for freehand 3D ultrasound. *J Ultras Med Biol*, Vol. 29, No. 11, pp. 1607-23.

Maintz JBA, & Viergever MA. (1998). A survey of medical image registration. *Medical Image Analysis*, Vol. 2, No. 1, pp. 1–36.

Martens V, Besirevic A, Shahin O, & Kleemann M. LapAssistent - computer assisted laparoscopic liver surgery. Conference Proceedings of Biomedizinischen Technik (BMT). Rostock, Germany, 2010.

Mårvik R, Langø T, Tangen GA, Andersen JON, Kaspersen JH, Ystgaard B, Sjølie E, Fougner R, Fjøsne HE, & Hernes TAN. (2004). Laparoscopic navigation pointer for 3-D image guided surgery. *Surg Endosc*, Vol. 18, No. 8, pp. 1242-8.

Mercier L, Langø T, Lindseth F, & Collins LD. (2005). A review of calibration techniques for freehand 3D ultrasound systems. *J Ultrasound Med Biol*, Vol. 31, No., pp. 449–71.

Nafis C, Jensen V, Beauregard L, & Anderson P. Method for estimating dynamic EM tracking accuracy of surgical navigation tools. In SPIE (Society of Photo-Optical Instrumentation Engineers) Medical Imaging 2006. San Diego, CA, USA, 2006. p. 16.

Nafis C, Jensen V, & von Jako R. Method for evaluating compatibility of commercial electromagnetic (EM) micro sensor tracking systems with surgical and imaging tables. In SPIE (Society of Photo-Optical Instrumentation Engineers) Medical Imaging 2008. San Diego, CA, USA, 2008. p. 15.

Nakada K, Nakamoto M, Sato Y, Konishi K, Hashizume M, & Tamura S. (2003). A Rapid Method for Magnetic Tracker Calibration Using a Magneto-optic Hybrid Tracker. *Lecture Notes in Computer Science (MICCAI)*, Vol. 2879, No., pp. 285-93.

Nakamoto M, Hirayama H, Sato Y, Konishi K, Kakeji Y, Hashizume M, & Tamura S. (2007). Recovery of respiratory motion and deformation of the liver using laparoscopic freehand 3D ultrasound system. *Medical Image Analysis*, Vol. 11, No. 5, pp. 429-42.

Nakamoto M, Nakada K, Sato Y, Konishi K, Hashizume M, & Tamura S. (2008). Intraoperative magnetic tracker calibration using a magneto-optic hybrid tracker for 3-D ultrasound-based navigation in laparoscopic surgery. *IEEE Trans Med Imaging*, Vol. 27, No. 2, pp. 255-70.

Phee SJ, & Yang K. (2010). Interventional navigation systems for treatment of unresectable liver tumor. *Med Biol Eng Comput*, Vol. 48, No., pp. 103-11.

Prager R, Rohling R, Gee A, & Berman L. (1998). Rapid calibration for 3-d freehand ultrasound. *Ultrasound Med Biol*, Vol. 24, No. 6, pp. 855–69.

Reinertsen I, Lindseth F, Unsgaard G, & Collins DL. (2007). Clinical validation of vessel based registration for correction of brain-shift. *Medical Image Analysis*, Vol. 11, No., pp. 673-84.

Richardson W, Stefanidis D, Mittal S, & Fanelli RD. (2010). SAGES guidelines for the use of laparoscopic ultrasound. *Surg Endosc*, Vol. 24, No., pp. 745–56.

Rutala WA. (1996). APIC guideline for selection and use of disinfectants. 1994, 1995, and 1996 APIC Guidelines Committee. *Am J Infect Control*, Vol. 24, No. 4, pp. 313-42.

Sato Y, Miyamoto M, Nakamoto M, Nakajima Y, Shimada M, Hashizume M, & Tamura S. (2001). 3D Ultrasound Image Acquisition Using a Magneto-optic Hybrid Sensor for Laparoscopic Surgery. *Lecture Notes in Computer Science (MICCAI)*, Vol. 2208, No., pp. 1151–3.

Scheuering M, Schenk A, Schneider A, Preim B, & Greiner G. (2003). Intraoperative Augmented Reality for Minimally Invasive Liver Interventions. *Proc SPIE*, Vol. 5029, No., pp. 407-17.

Schicho K, Figl M, Donat M, Birkfellner W, Seemann R, Wagner A, Bergmann H, & Ewers R. (2005). Stability of miniature electromagnetic tracking systems. *Phys Med Biol*, Vol. 50, No., pp. 2089–98.

Schmerber S, & Chassat F. (2001). Accuracy evaluation of a CAS system: laboratory protocol and results with 6D localizers, and clinical experiences in otorhinolaryngology. *Comput Aided Surg*, Vol. 6, No., pp. 1–13.

Shahidi R, Bax MR, & Maurer CR. (2002). Implementation, Calibration and Accuracy Testing of an Image Enhanced Endoscopy System. *IEEE Trans Med Imaging*, Vol. 21, No., pp. 1524-35.

Sindram D, McKillop IH, Martinie JB, & Iannitti DA. (2010). Novel 3-d laparoscopic magnetic ultrasound image guidance for lesion targeting. *Journal of Hepato-Pancreato Bilary Association*, Vol. 12, No. 10, pp. 709-16.

Solberg OV, Langø T, Tangen GA, Mårvik R, Ystgaard B, Rethy A, & Hernes TAN. (2009). Navigated ultrasound in laparoscopic surgery. *Minimally Invasive Therapy and Allied Technologies (MITAT)*, Vol. 18, No. 1, pp. 36-53.

Solberg OV, Lindseth F, Torp H, Blake RE, & Hernes TAN. (2007). Freehand 3D Ultrasound Reconstruction Algorithms—A Review. *J Ultras Med Biol*, Vol. 33, No. 7, pp. 991-1009.

Unsgaard G, Gronningsaeter A, Ommedal S, & Hernes TAN. (2002). Brain operations guided by real time 2D ultrasound New possibilities due to improved image quality. *Neurosurgery*, Vol. 51, No., pp. 402-12.

Unsgaard G, Rygh OM, Selbekk T, Müller TB, Kolstad F, Lindseth F, & Hernes TAN. (2006). Intra-operative 3D ultrasound in neurosurgery. *Acta Neurochirurgica*, Vol. 148, No. 3, pp. 235-53.

Våpenstad C, Rethy A, Langø T, Selbekk T, Ystgaard B, Hernes TA, & Marvik R. (2010). Laparoscopic ultrasound: a survey of its current and future use, requirements, and integration with navigation technology. *Surg Endosc*, Vol. 24, No. 12, pp. 2944-53.

Wilheim D, Feussner H, Schneider A, & Harms J. (2003). Electromagnetically navigated laparoscopic ultrasound. *Surg Technol Int*, Vol. 11, No., pp. 50-4.

Wilson E, Yaniv Z, & Zhang H. A hardware and software protocol for the evaluation of electromagnetic tracker accuracy in the clinical environment: a multi-center study. Proc in Medical Imaging 2007: Visualization and Image-Guided Procedures (SPIE). San Diego, USA, 2007. p. 65092T.

Yamakawa K, Naito S, & Azuma K. (1958). Laparoscopic diagnosis of the intraabdominal organs. *Jpn J Gastroenterol*, Vol. 55, No., pp. 741-7.

7

Single Port Laparoscopic Surgery

Carus Thomas
Department of General, Visceral and Trauma Surgery,
Center for Minimally Invasive Surgery,
Klinikum Bremen-Ost/ Gesundheit Nord GmbH,
Germany

1. Introduction

In the last two decades, almost every operation in the abdominal and thoracic cavity - from a simple diagnostic laparoscopy to esophagectomy – has been successfully performed by minimally invasive technique. In interventions such as cholecystectomy for symptomatic cholelithiasis or sigmoid resection for recurrent diverticulitis the laparoscopic, minimally invasive procedure is now considered standard.

It should not go unmentioned that Erich Mühe from Böblingen/ Germany performed the first laparoscopic cholecystectomy worldwide in 1985 with his "Galloskop", a multi channel single-port trocar. (1) Giuseppe Navarra from Italy published 1997 his "one-wound-cholecystectomy" with standard trocars introduced through one skin incision. (2)

Since the first transvaginal NOTES cholecystectomy (natural orifice transluminal endoscopic surgery) in 2007 (3) special interest lays in minimizing the access trauma to reach a (nearly) scarless surgery. In 2008 the first special trocars to perform a laparoscopic operation through one small incision became available (single port laparoscopic surgery). From this time "standard" laparoscopy via 3 – 4 incisions had to compete with NOTES and single port laparoscopic surgery.

In a very short time multidisciplinary applications were developed and are still expanding. Single port laparoscopic surgery has potential advantages for e.g. postoperative pain, wound infections and cosmesis. This chapter will give an overview of technology, handling and clinical application.

2. Single port laparoscopic surgery

In single port laparoscopic surgery the surgeon operates through a single access point, usually the patient's umbilicus. Several expressions are used to describe these procedures:

SPL	single-port laparoscopy
SPT	single-port technique
SPA	single-port(al) access
SPICES	single-port incisionless conventional equipment-utilizing surgery

SILS	single incision laparoscopic surgery
OPUS	one-port umbilical surgery
TUE	transumbilical endoscopic surgery
LESS	laparoscopic-endoscopic single site
NOTUS	natural orifice transumbilical surgery
E-NOTES	embryonic
NOTES	(= umbilical access)

The term "SILS" is registered by the company Covidien, "LESS" is usually used by the company Olympus. We generally use the neutral term "SPL" for single port laparoscopy.

2.1 Special devices and instruments

To perform single port procedures successfully many surgeons use special devices and instruments. There is an increasing number of products for both groups.

2.1.1 Special trocars and access ports

Single port access starts with a 15 - 20 mm skin incision in the umbilicus or at the lower circumference of the umbilicus. (Figure 1) For special indications like e.g. SPL-IPOM incisional hernia repair the access is positioned on the right or left side of the patient's abdomen.

After dissecting the subcutaneous tissue and opening the ventral fascia, the rectus muscles are pulled to both sides with Langenbeck hooks. The posterior sheath and the peritoneum are pulled upwards and opened by scissors. The Langenbeck hooks are placed under the peritoneum (Figure 2). If there are local adhesions, they can be dissected by finger or sharply under direct visual control.

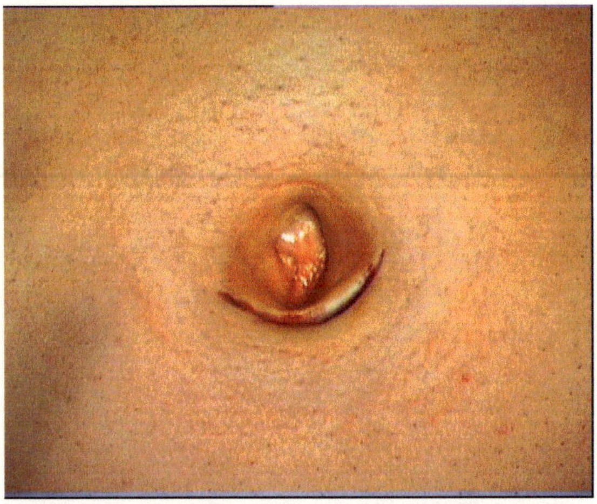

Fig. 1. Subumbilical incision for single port laparoscopy

A special single port device can than be introduced through this access. Starting in 2008 with the single-use TriPort system (Advanced Surgical) many different devices were developed in the last years. Examples for single-use devices are TriPort and QuadPort (now: Olympus), SILS-Port (Covidien), GelPOINT (Applied Medical) and Uni-X (Pnavel).

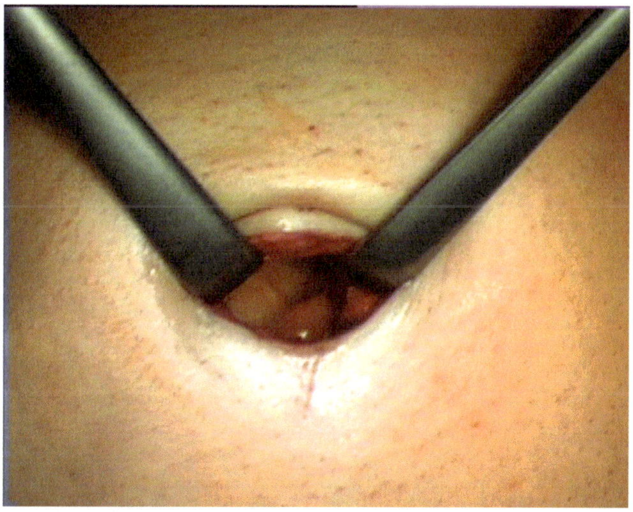

Fig. 2. Open access to the abdominal cavity

Reusable single port devices were developed by Karl Storz company with the X-Cone and EndoCone.

In the following examples are shown how to handle these special devices.

Usage of the SILS-Port (Covidien)

The SILS-Port is a flexible device for single-use with three open channels for the insertion of 5 - 12 mm trocars and one channel with a tube for gas supply. The widening at both ends allows a secure fit under the peritoneum and prevents dislocation into the abdomen. (Figure 3)

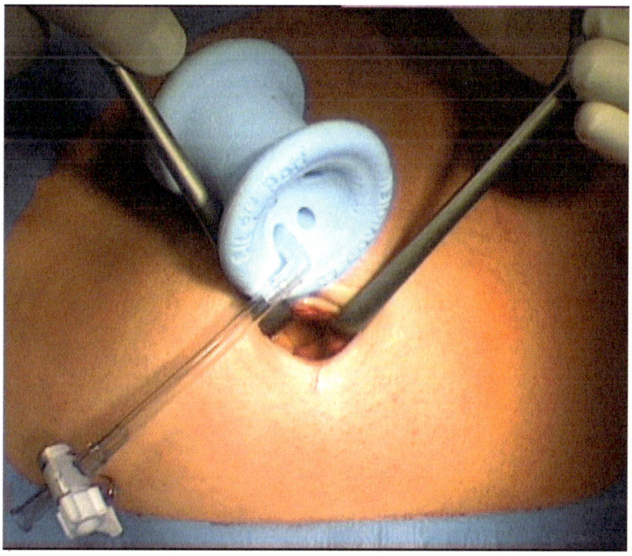

Fig. 3. Shape of the SILS-Port

By pushing the lower widening together, the SILS-Port can be easily pushed into the opening. If the incision is smaller than 20 mm, it is helpful to use a lubricant. (Figure 4)

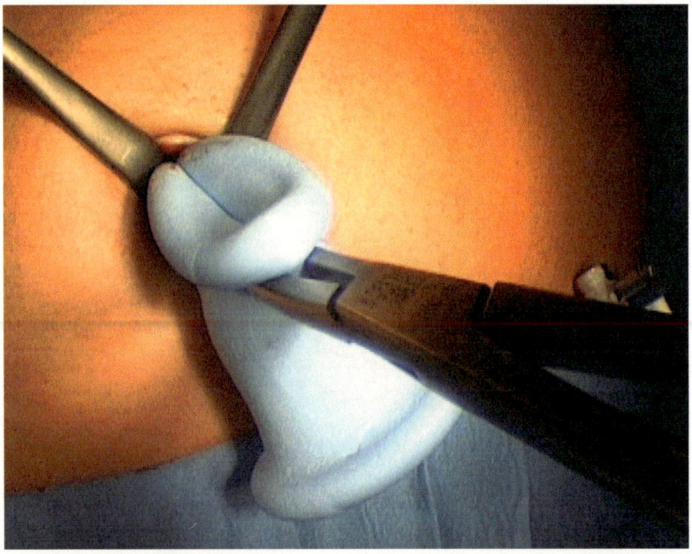

Fig. 4. Introducing the SILS-Port

After correct placement gas supply is connected and three trocars are gently pushed into the channels. We normally use one flexible 5 mm trocar for use of a curved instrument, one straight 5 mm trocar for a standard instrument and another 5 (or 10) mm trocar for the optic. (Figure 5). You can as well use only straight trocars, single-use or reusable from 5 to 12 mm diameter size.

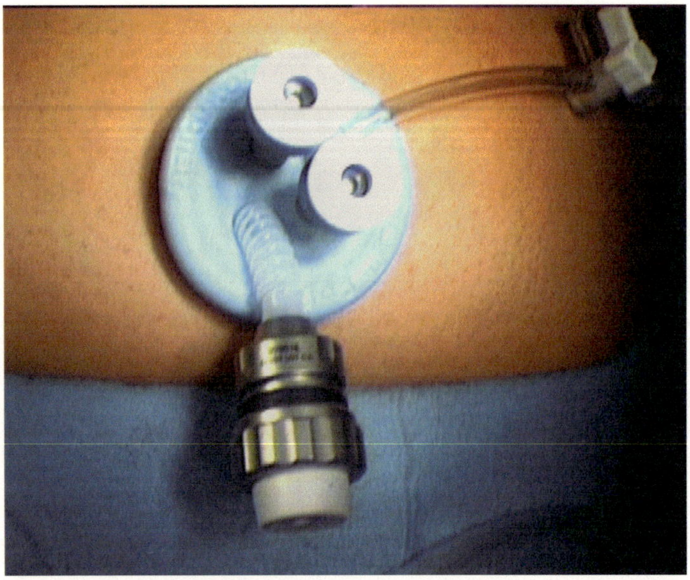

Fig. 5. SILS-Port with 3 trocars and gas supply

Usage of the TriPort (Olympus)

The TriPort device is an example for a single-use single port system, which consists of two (or more) pieces. A flexible tube is introduced into the abdominal cavity while a head piece is mounted on the tube. (Figure 6)

The tube is than pulled upwards until the inner ring of the tube touches the peritoneum. (Figure 7)

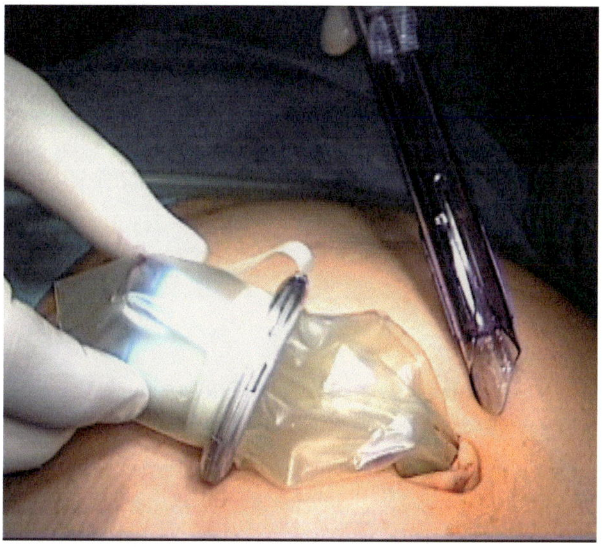

Fig. 6. TriPort with inserted tube and introducer

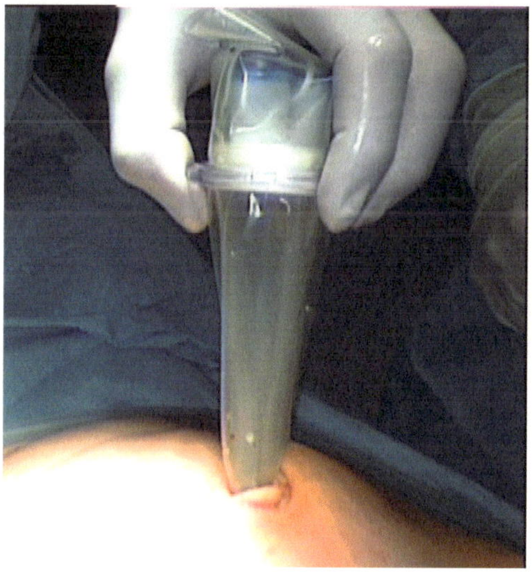

Fig. 7. Tensioned tube and head piece

The head piece is pushed down to abdominal wall to give enough tension for a stable fixation. (Figure 8)

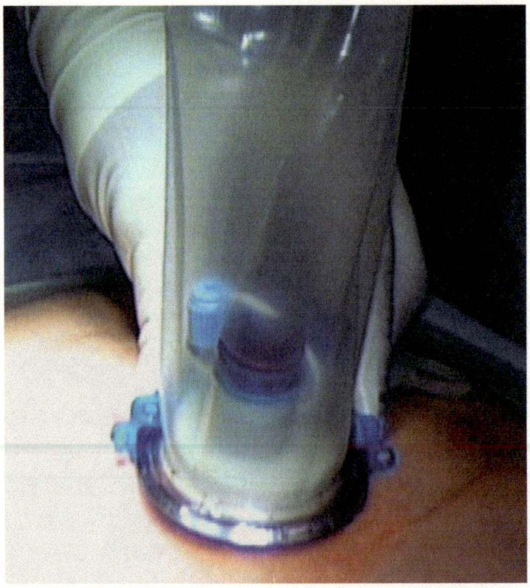

Fig. 8. Head piece in final position

This position is held by mounting two brackets. The ready system has one port for gas supply and 3 ports with silicone valves for the instruments. (Figure 9)

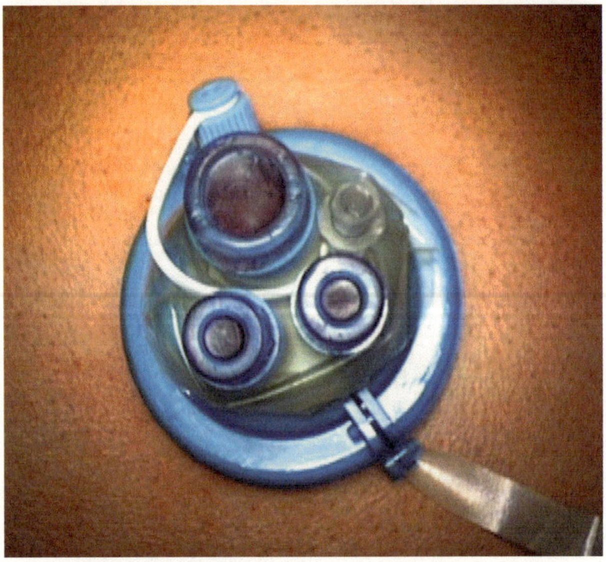

Fig. 9. TriPort with 3 valves and gas supply

Usage of the X-Cone (Karl Storz)

The X-Cone represents a reusable system, which consists of 2 specially shaped metal hooks and one rubber cap with 5 valves. The metal hooks are shell-shaped at the top and build a semi-circular tube at the bottom. The two half-tubes are plugged together and can be easily introduced through the incision. (Figure 10)

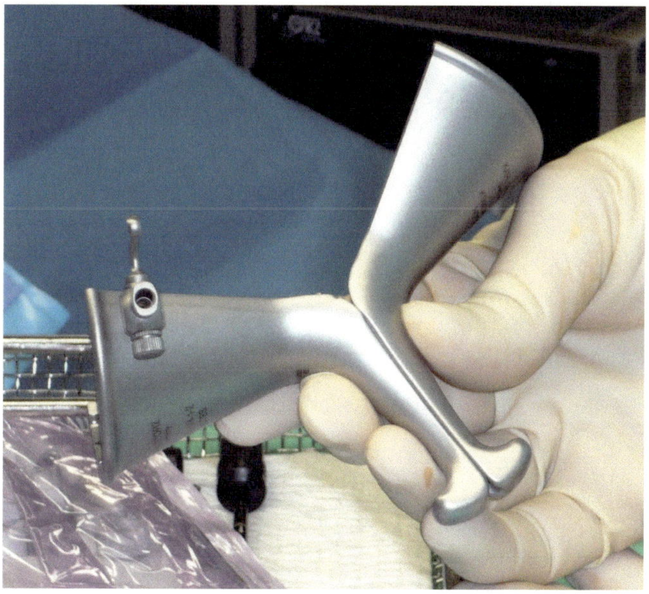

Fig. 10. X-Cone with closed half-tubes

When the half-tubes are inside the abdominal cavity, the upper portions are folded together. They form a ring and bring the lower portions in an X-shape. (Figure 11)

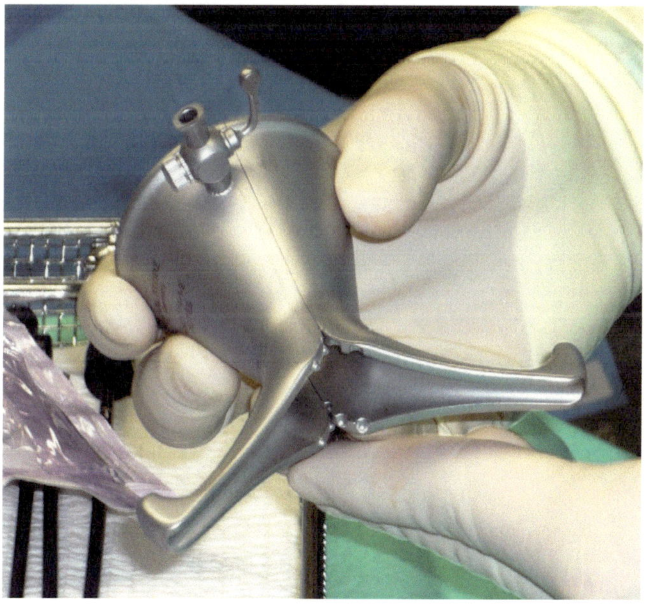

Fig. 11. X-Cone with closed upper portions in X-shape

Finally a rubber cap with 5 valves for one optic and up to 4 instruments is mounted on the ring. The rubber cap has to be replaced when it is worn while the metal parts can be used hundreds of times. (Figure 12)

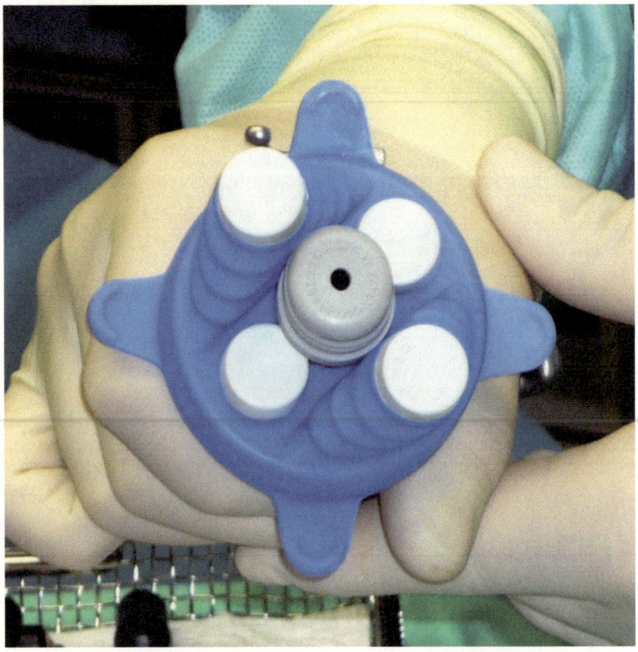

Fig. 12. X-Cone with rubber cap and 5 valves

To pull out the resected organs, the rubber cap is removed for an easy access. (Figure 13)

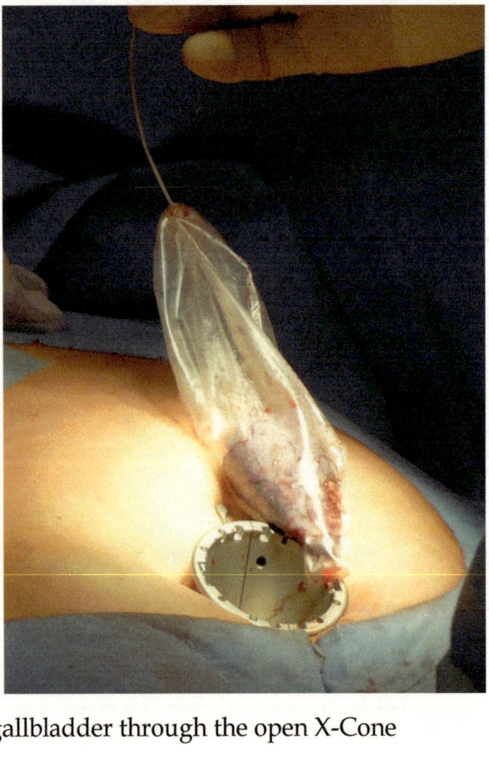

Fig. 13. Extraction of a gallbladder through the open X-Cone

Due to their construction the systems have specific advantages and disadvantages. A rigid shaft like with the X-Cone leads in comparison to the flexible ports to a tighter fit in the abdominal wall with a good gas tightness. The mobility of the instruments shafts is a bit more restricted. A very flexible approach as the TriPort makes the introduction easier but may lead to slight dislocation and corresponding gas loss especially in long during operations. The SILS-Port takes a middle position with a good stability and enough flexibility.

The development of single-port devices is still in the beginning. Many other will follow with its specific characteristics, advantages and disadvantages. Currently the surgeon chooses the type of single-port device according to his personal experiences.

2.1.2 Special instruments

When a single port device is used, one or two working instruments are introduced in a parallel way close to the optic. The surgeon's hands and the optics interfere with each other and restrict the mobility.

Two paths are followed to facilitate this problem: instruments which are bendable inside the abdominal cavity or curved instruments extend the distance between hands and optic. The same effect can be achieved by an optic with a movable lens or a bendable shaft.

One example of a curved instrument is shown in Figure 14. It is constructed with a standard shaft, which allows a full 360° rotation, and a curved tip. The view is not limited by parallel instrument tips and triangulation is much easier. Additionally the "knee" of the tip helps to keep other organs away from the preparation zone.

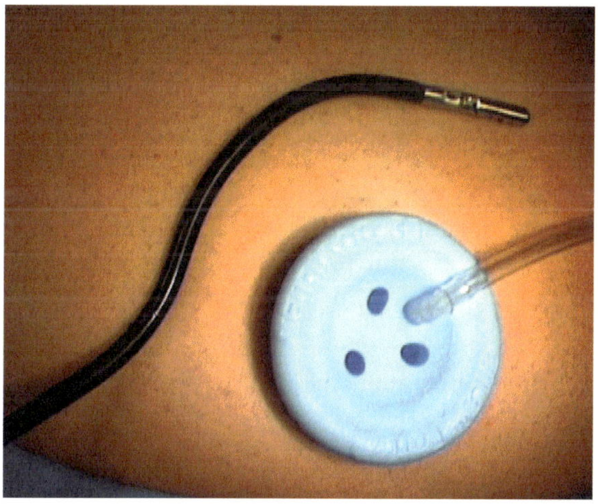

Fig. 14. Curved single-port instrument (forceps by Carus)

2.1.3 Optical devices

In standard or "conventional" laparoscopy, optical devices with a 0° or 30° lens are normally used. The instruments do not touch the optic, because the working trocars are far enough away from the optic. There will be no disturbing interference between surgeon's hands and the optic.

In single port laparoscopy the proximity between hands and optic represent the greatest problem. In addition to using special instruments an optic with a movable lens or a bendable shaft is very helpful.

By turning the lens to 60 or more degrees, the camera-holding hand can be moved down and gives space for the working hands. (Figure 15)

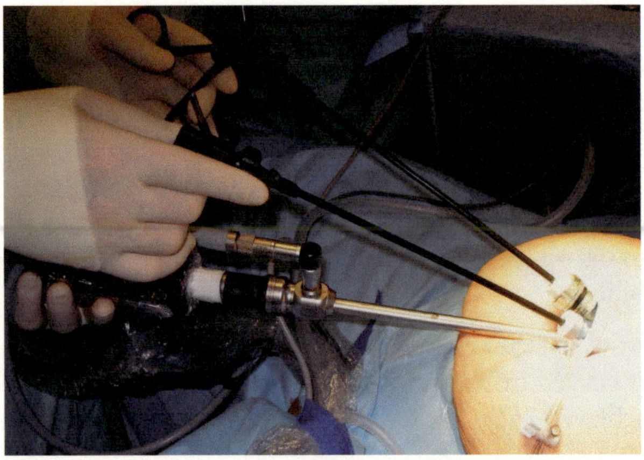

Fig. 15. Single-port optic with movable lens in 60° position during single port cholecystectomy

2.2 Clinical application

Modern techniques allow laparoscopic surgeons to perform complex operations with great certainty. Numerous studies (4) demonstrate the benefits to the patient by a lower need for analgetics, partially reduced perioperative complications, a better cosmetic result and a rapid convalescence. (5, 6)

The spectrum of single port laparoscopic surgery (SPLS) is broad and includes operations from simple diagnostic laparoscopy to gastrectomy or liver resection. SPLS does not lead to an expansion of existing spectrum but offers the chance to further minimize the access trauma with a new technique and ergonomy. The implementation of SPLS requires excellent laparoscopic skills.

In the following some elective operations, which are increasingly performed in SPLS, are described.

2.2.1 Single port laparoscopic cholecystectomy

Up to now single port laparoscopic cholecystectomy is the most commonly practised single port procedure. Pubmed literature search shows 136 results for "single port laparoscopic cholecystectomy" and 55 results for "SILS cholecystectomy" on July 21st 2011. (e.g. 6, 7, 8, 9)

After umbilical access the optic (5 or 10 mm) and 2 instruments are introduced through a single port device. The gallbladder is lifted with the left hand; preparation is performed by the right hand of the surgeon. (Figure 16)

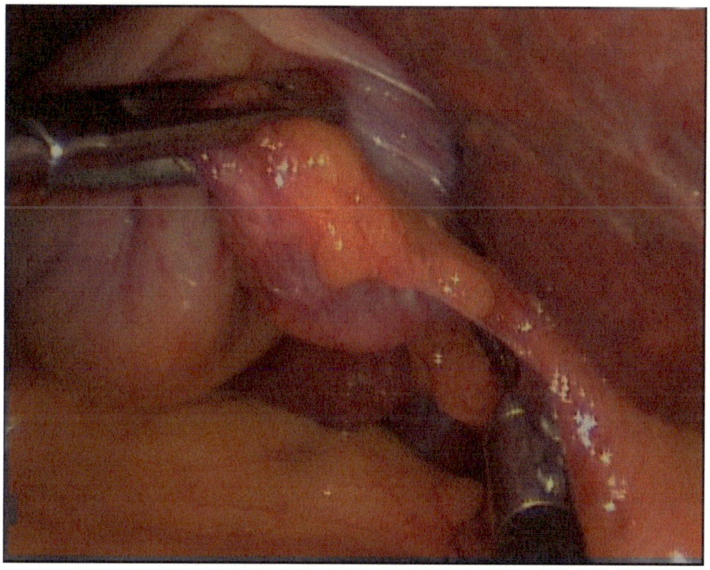

Fig. 16. Single port preparation with curved forceps (left) and straight dissector (right)

Because of the more difficult triangulation in single port technique exposure of the Calot triangle is challenging. It requires much more accuracy than in "conventional" laparoscopy. (Figure 17)

After adequate exposure of cystic duct and cystic artery, both structures are dissected between metal or absorbable clips. The gallbladder is lifted with the curved forceps, the resection can than be easily done with an ultrasonic hook. (Figure 18)

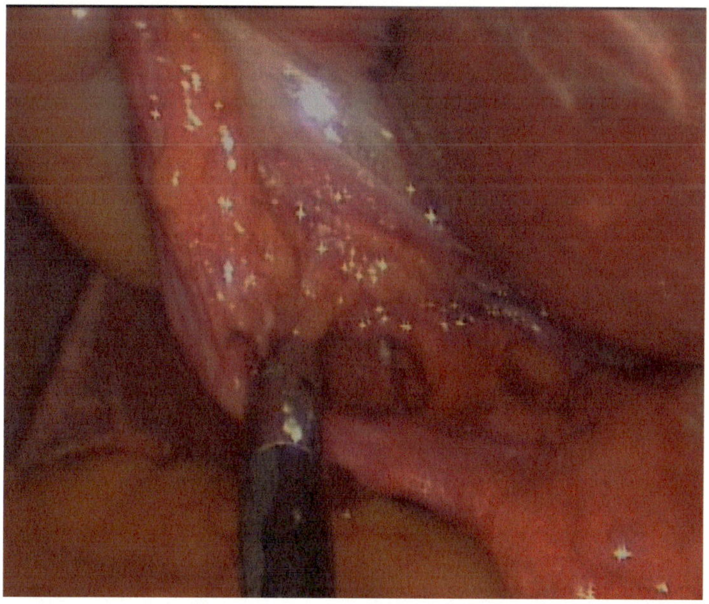

Fig. 17. Exposure of the cystic duct and its confluence with the common bile duct

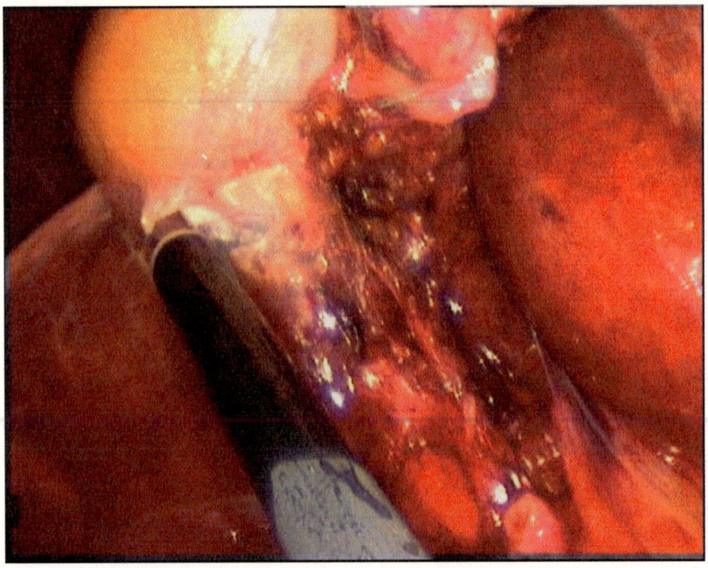

Fig. 18. Resection of the gall bladder with ultrasonic hook

After complete resection the gallbladder is put into an endobag and pulled out of the abdominal cavity together via the single port device. (Figure 19) The use of an intraabdominal drain is optional.

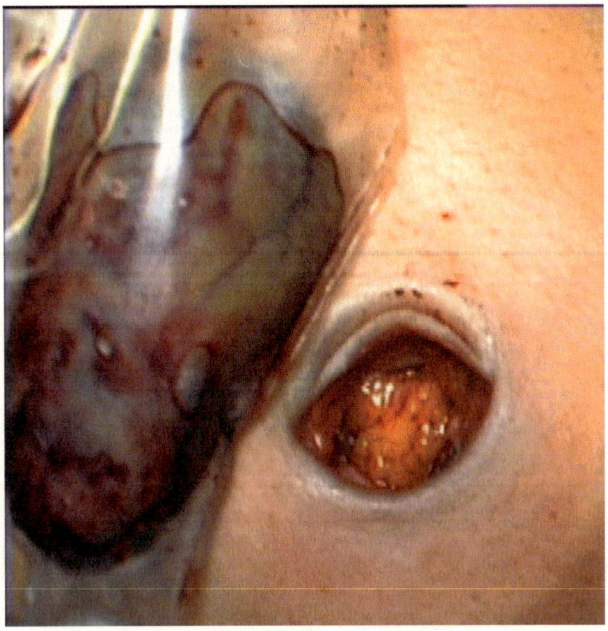

Fig. 19. Removal of the gallbladder via the single port incision

Some surgeons use extra tools like an auxiliary 3 – 5 mm trocar in the right upper abdomen or transabdominal sutures to lift the gallbladder and facilitate the single port procedure. We prefer "pure" single port operations with only one incision to offer the patient the least traumatic access.

Previously published studies show similar good results for single port and "conventional" laparoscopic cholecystectomy.

The small incision for single port access leads to an almost invisible scar and less postoperative pain. (5, 6, 8, 9) Disadvantages of single port cholecystectomy are a prolonged operation time (plus 10 - 45 minutes), more difficult exposure of important anatomic structures and higher costs. (10, 11)

2.2.2 Single port laparoscopic unroofing of liver cysts

Several publications (e.g. 12, 13) describe the successful laparoscopic unroofing of symptomatic, non-parasitic liver cysts - especially in segments VII and VIII. The first single-port fenestration of a liver cyst was described in 2010 by Mantke et al. (14). We use the single port access as our standard operation for symptomatic liver cysts which are close to the liver surface.

The access and the instruments are similar to single port cholecystectomy. Using an optic with a flexible lens helps to expose structures on the lateral aspect of the right liver lobe. (Figures 20 and 21)

The unroofing and resection of the anterior cystic wall can be easily done with an ultrasonic hook or scissors. (Figure 22)

The resected tissue (Figure 23) is put into an endobag and removed via the single port device.

Although there are less than 5 publications up to now - mostly single case descriptions - single port technique could be a safe and feasible procedure for surgical therapy of symptomatic liver cysts in selected patients.

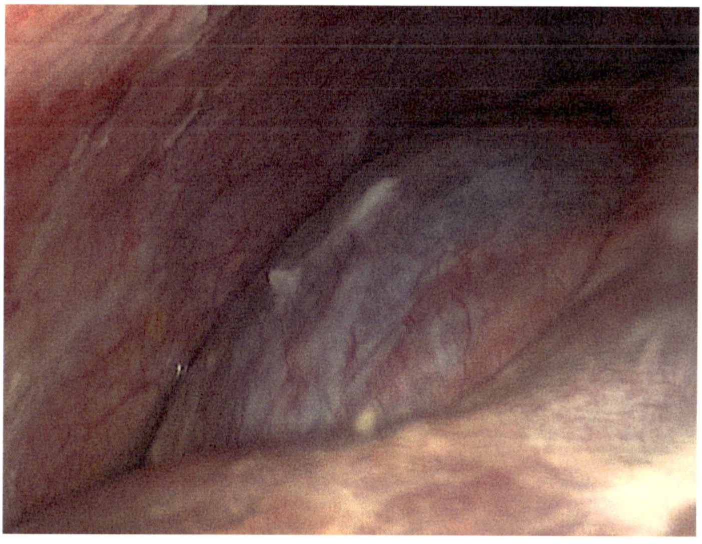

Fig. 20. Symptomatic liver cyst (segment VII): 0° view

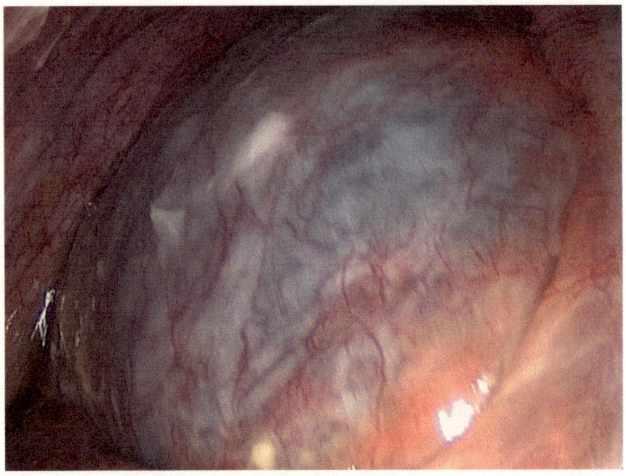

Fig. 21. Symptomatic liver cyst (segment VII): 60° view

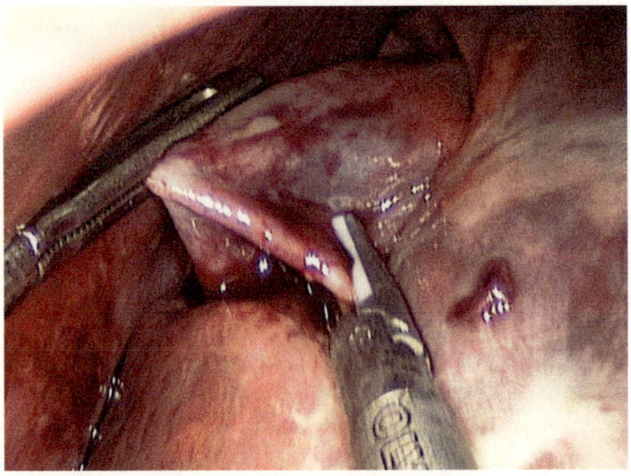

Fig. 22. Resection of a symptomatic liver cyst (segment VII)

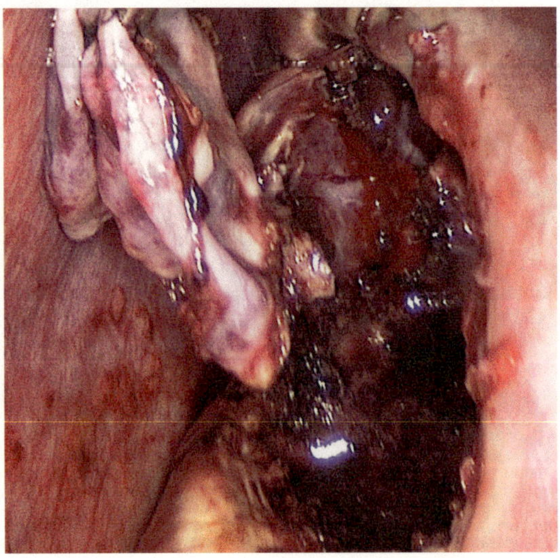

Fig. 23. Unroofed liver cyst with resected anterior wall

2.2.3 Single port colorectal operations

All kinds of colorectal operations have been successfully performed in single port technique. The spectrum reaches from "simple" colostomy to proctocolectomy and J-pouch reconstruction (15).

More than 150 single port colonic procedures are published with a monthly increasing number. The most frequent operation is - like in "conventional" laparoscopic surgery - the sigmoid resection for recurrent diverticulitis or small sigmoid cancers. The technique of preparation, dissection, resection and anastomosis does not differ from standard laparoscopic sigmoid resection. Handling and lifting of a large or elongated sigma is more difficult with a subjective feeling of a "missing hand".

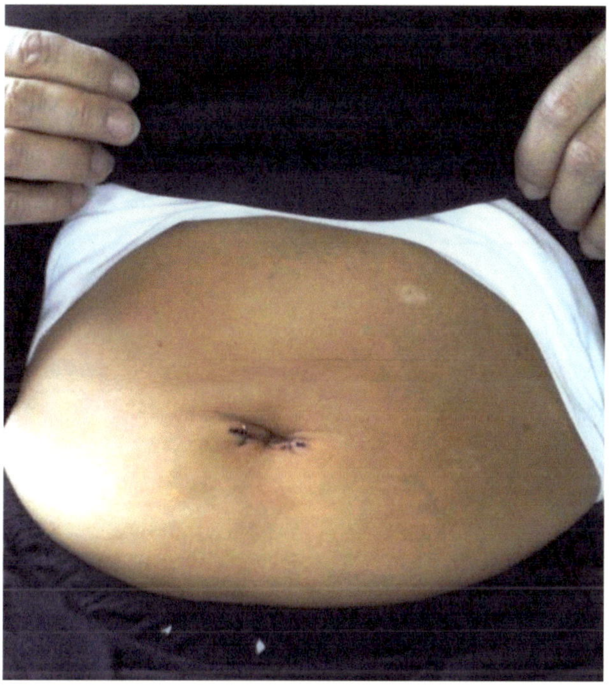

Fig. 24. 2nd day after single port laparoscopic sigmoid resection

There are no significant differences in colorectal surgery between single port or multi port access, conversion rate from single to multi port access lies between 5 - 10 %. (15, 16)

Although the umbilical incision has to be 3 - 4 or sometimes even up to 6 centimetres for the removal of the bowel, the cosmetic result and the almost painless postoperative course are impressing. (5, 15) Figure 24 shows a 56 years old female patient on 2nd day after single port laparoscopic sigmoid resection for recurrent diverticulitis.

2.2.4 Summary of clinical applications

Potential advantages and disadvantages of single port laparoscopic surgery are listed in following table 1.

Laparoscopic procedure	Effect of single port technique
Diagnostic laparoscopy	Higher costs by single-use instruments
Adhesiolysis	Limited use in case of complex adhesions
Appendectomy	Higher costs by single-use instruments
Cholecystectomy	Safe and effective, better cosmetic result, difficult in advanced inflammation
Inguinal herniotomy	Suitable for transabdominal technique difficult for extraperitoneal technique
Fundoplication	Very difficult when using intracorporeal Suturing technique
Gastric sleeve and wedge resections	Suitable when using linear staplers
Gastric bypass	Limited use by complexity of procedure
Pancreatic resections	Suitable for left resections, limitation for complex resections
Colorectal procedures	Suitable for uncomplicated resections
Splenectomy	Difficult in splenomegaly
Gynecological and urological procedures	Suitable for non-complex operations

Table 1. Clinical applications of single port laparoscopic surgery

3. Conclusion

Single port laparoscopic surgery offers the possibility to further minimize the access trauma to the abdominal wall. Recent publications and our own experience have shown that the new method is safe and efficient. For the surgeon it is technically much more demanding to perform a complex laparoscopic procedure via a single port trocar than via 3 – 5 trocars. The patient may benefit from reduced postoperative pain, better cosmetic results and a faster recovery.

A comparison between single port and "conventional" laparoscopic surgery is shown in table 2.

Actually single port laparoscopic surgery shows disadvantages concerning the limitation for complex operations and higher costs by using a single port special trocar.

As with any new technology a further development of instruments and surgical skills is necessary to overcome the limitations. With a wider spread extra costs will decrease.

To show significant advantages compared to "conventional" laparoscopic surgery, randomized studies are necessary.

	Single port laparoscopic surgery	"Conventional" laparoscopic surgery
First access	Special technique	Verres needle or open
Optic	Always via single port	Different positions possible through working trocars
Triangulation	Limited, difficult	Almost unlimited, easy
Dissection and resection	Difficult in complex operations	Easy by variable trocar positions
Handling	Difficult, feeling of "missing hand"	Easy by variable trocar positions
Suitable for complex operations	Limited use	Less limitations
Wound care	Only one incision, scar almost invisible	Several incisions
Postoperative complications	Very rare	Very rare
Cosmetic result	Very good	Good
Costs	Extra costs by single port trocar	No extra costs
Significant benefit	Not known	Not known

Table 2. Comparison between single port and "conventional" laparoscopic surgery

4. References

[1] Mühe, E. (1992). Laparoscopic cholecystectomy follow up. Endoscopy 24:754-758

[2] Navarra, G.; Pozza, E.; Occhionorelli, S. et al. (1997). One-wound laparoscopic cholecystectomy. Br J Surg 84:695

[3] Marescaux, J.; Dallemagne, B.; Perretta, S. (2007). Surgery without scars: a report of transluminal cholecystectomy in a human being. Arch Surg 142(9):823-826

[4] Schwenk, W.; Haase, O.; Neudecker, J.; Müller, J.M. (2005). Short term benefits for laparoscopic colorectal resection. Cochrane Database Syst Rev. 20(3):CD003145

[5] Carus, T. (2010). Single-port technique in laparoscopic surgery. Chirurg 81:431-439

[6] Langwieler, T.E.; Back, M. (2011). Single-port access cholecystectomy. Current status. Chirurg 82:406-410

[7] McGregor, C.G.; Sodergren, M.H.; Aslanyan, A.; Wright, V.J. et al. (2011). Evaluating systemic stress response in single port vs. multi-port laparoscopic cholecystectomy. J Gastrointest Surg. 15(4):614-622

[8] Hernandez, J.M.; Morton, C.A.; Ross, S. et al. (2009). Laparoendoscopic single site cholecystectomy : the first 100 patients. Am Surg 75(8):681-685
[9] Langwieler, T.E.; Nimmesgern, T.; Back, M. (2009). Singleport access in laparoscopic cholecystectomy. Surg endosc 23(5):1138-1141
[10] Aprea, G.; Coppola Bottazzi, E.; Guida, F.; Masone, S.; Persico, G. (2011). Laparoendoscopic single site (LESS) versus classic video-laparoscopic cholecystectomy : a randomized prospective study. J Surg Res. 166(2):e109-112
[11] Ma, J.; Cassera, M.A.; Spaun, G.O.; Hammill, C.W.; Hansen, P.D.; Aliabadi-Wahle, S. (2011). Randomized controlled trial comparing single-port laparoscopic cholecystectomy and four-port laparoscopic cholecystectomy. Ann Surg. 254(1):22-27
[12] Tagaya, N.; Nemoto, T.; Kubota, K. (2003). Long-term results of laparoscopic unroofing of symptomatic solitary nonparasitic hepatic cysts. Surg Laparosc Endosc Percutan Tech. 13(2):76-79
[13] Weber, T.; Sendt, W.; Scheele, J. (2004). Laparoscopic unroofing of nonparasitic liver cysts within segments VII and VIII: technical considerations. J Laparoendosc Adv Surg Tech A. 14(1):37-42
[14] Mantke, R.; Wicht, S. (2010). Single-port liver cyst fenestration combined with Single-port laparoscopic cholecystectomy using completely reusable instruments. Surg Laparosc Endosc Percutan Tech 20:28-30
[15] Vestweber, V.; Straub, E.; Kaldowski, B. et al. (2011). Single-port colonic surgery. Techniques and indications. Chirurg 82:411-418
[16] Diana, M.; Dhumane, P.; Cahill, R.A.; Mortensen, N.; Leroy, J.; Marescaux, J. (2011). Minimal invasive single-site surgery in colorectal procedures: Current state of the art. 7(1):52-60

Part 4

Pediatric Procedures

8

Laparoscopic Approach as an Alternative Option in Treatment of Pediatric Inguinal Hernia

B. Haluk Güvenç
Professor of Pediatric Surgery,
Turkey

1. Introduction

Inguinal hernia is the most common and prominent surgical entity among all congenital anomalies, constituting more than 15% of total pediatric surgical cases. Inguinal hernia is directly linked to the descent of the developing gonads in children. A patent processus vaginalis, which precedes an inguinal hernia, is a diverticulum of the peritoneum, formed during gonadal descent around the 12th week of gestation. This blind-ending, celomic epithelium layered sac is generally obliterated after the testicular migration is completed. A failure during the obliteration process may develop an inguinal hernia or communicating hydrocele[1-3].

In children, the bowel follows the course of the processus vaginalis through the internal ring, lateral to the inferior epigastric vessels forming an indirect inguinal hernia. The diagnosis of hernia can be made during physical examination when organs such as bowel or ovary protrude into the sac, or can be based on a classic description by the parents or a referring physician. On the other hand, a communicating hydrocele should also be considered as a hernia, and repair is indicated regardless of the age. Hydroceles that develop after birth are more likely to be associated with a patent processus vaginalis that is less likely to close[3].

The surgical repair of a pediatric inguinal hernia should take place in a timely manner to eliminate any risk of incarceration. The classic open repair is performed through a skin incision, made in the inguinal crease overlying the internal ring. Scarpa's fascia and the external oblique aponeurosis are opened. In males, the cremasteric fibers are bluntly dissected until the sac can be seen. The sac is then gently separated from the cord structures, divided, dissected to the level of the internal ring, and ligated at this level. In females, the sac is dissected to the level of the internal ring and ligated. Reconstruction of the inguinal ring is not routinely necessary[1, 2].

Data from surgical practice and autopsy studies suggest a strong likelihood of bilateralism in children with a unilateral presentation. The increase in cost, the unpleasant experience of additional operative risk and mental trauma for the patient accompanied by the anxiety of the parents that may result from a metachronous hernia, have led surgeons to adopt a policy of routine bilateral exploration [4, 5]. Bilateral inguinal exploration may be justified in patients known to be at higher risk for bilateral hernias or at increased operative risk, such as premature infants or patients with bladder extrophy, ascites, cystic fibrosis, ventriculoperitoneal shunts, peritoneal dialysis catheters, or connective tissue disorders. In the meantime, due to fact that the rate of patency decreases with age and the accumulation of data showing a higher risk of damage to the vas deferens and gonad during negative exploration, proponents had to restrict bilateral exploration according to the age and sex of the child and the presenting side[6-15]. The author believes that a "prophylactic" contralateral exploration in children presenting with unilateral hernia is unjustified.

2. The search for contralateral patent processus vaginalis

The introduction of laparoscopic intervention is a milestone in understanding the concept of contemporary pediatric inguinal hernia repair. The debate amongst the proponents and opponents of bilateral inguinal exploration in children, is about to end. The accumulated data concerning the presence and fate of patent processus vaginalis (PPV) about the incidence, relation to age or presenting side and timing of obliteration will be of historic importance in the near future. The true incidence of bilateral hernia however, is still unclear.

Searching through the published data, we may see that the given incidence of a contralateral inguinal hernia is as high as 57% to 85% according to the proponents of bilateral exploration [16, 17]. The incidence of a PPV on the other hand, is reported as 80% in the first 2 months of life, steadily decreasing over the next 2 years[18, 19]. Nakayama and Rowe stating that in about 60% of infants, a contralateral PPV may accompany a clinically presenting unilateral inguinal hernia report a similar rough estimation. One-third of these anatomic patencies is expected to be obliterated within 2 years, one-third is expected to develop into a subsequent hernia, and the remaining one-third will be clinically silent [20, 21]. Published series concerning adult patients does support the estimated incidence. Adult patients without a clinical hernia, present with a surprisingly high number (12 %) of true indirect PPVs, with a defect of around 3 cm seen through the telescope[22-24]. Again, the controversy remains; some authors [23] do not recommend prophylactic repair of such an asymptomatic defect, while others do recommend simultaneous repair[22].

Studies investigating the most suitable method in evaluating the contralateral side have been an important topic for many years, since the reported incidence of a developing contralateral hernia is as high as 30%[25]. A rather recent meta-analysis by Miltenburg et al. discloses the rate of a metachronous hernia as 7 - 11 %, covering over 13.000 children undergoing unilateral repair[26]. Consideration of all processus vaginalis' as a future clinically significant hernia may attribute to the discrepancy between figures. Contemporary use of ultrasound has revolutionized near precise preoperative diagnosis of a contralateral inguinal hernia when compared to a number of (now historical) tests such as herniography, the Goldstein procedure, and use of Bakes dilators[27]. This precision though has been mastered through hard-earned lessons, in search for a less invasive method following introduction of diagnostic laparoscopy in the early 1990's[28-34]. Diagnostic laparoscopic evaluation of the contralateral inguinal ring is regarded as a reliable method, with a sensitivity of 99.4% and a specificity of 99.5%[35]. The method is accurate, fast, safe, and effective in reducing negative explorations, avoiding the small risk of incarceration of a metachronous hernia as well as the cost and anxiety of a second operation; it is easily learned and requires no additional capital outlay in hospitals already performing laparoscopic surgery.

2.1 Diagnostic laparoscopy

The decisive step of performing a diagnostic laparoscopy aids the surgeon in solving the dilemma, the postoperative complications from an unnecessary inguinal exploration or a missed metachronous hernia. It is a promising step taken forward with respect to the surgical precision achieved through enhanced visualization, magnification and ability to limit collateral damage by minimizing invasion. An additional benefit is the ability to detect all forms of (indirect, direct, combined, recurrent, and incarcerated) hernias(19).

The suggested techniques of diagnostic laparoscopy for evaluating a contralateral patency mainly include three primary methods. The open infraumbilical approach has the advantage of permitting a direct view of the internal ring and better correlation of the two sides(28, 30-33). To avoid a second incision and eliminate the risk of intra-abdominal visceral injury associated with trocar placement, the already-opened ipsilateral hernia sac is used in the second method, referred to as the "nonpuncture" technique(29, 30, 32-34). This technique requires understanding of the view through an angled telescope, since a peritoneal veil or the median umbilical fold may obscure the direct view in some patients (36, 37). This examination is even harder in small babies, as the distance between the two internal rings is very short. The placement of the trocar is safe, but it is not possible to proceed when the hernia sac is too narrow or friable. The third technique is the "inline" method, in which a telescope is introduced through a 14- or 16-gauge catheter placed in line with the contralateral internal ring and the abdomen is insufflated through the ipsilateral sac. This technique has the advantage of providing a direct view and enables measurement of the depth of any processus vaginalis(38, 39). As for measuring the depth, a 2.7 mm 30° angled Hopkins rod lens is inserted to its maximum depth in the internal ring, and then the shaft of the scope where it entered the port is marked. A second mark is made after withdrawing the scope until the tip is at the internal ring. One can proceed with laparoscopy with this method when the ipsilateral hernia sac is too narrow or friable to insert a trocar. This technique means a second wound and may carry a risk of injury to the bowel and abdominal wall vessels. Depending on the chosen technique, the surgeon may utilize a range of rigid or flexible telescopes from 1.2 mm to 5 mm with an optic range of 0° to 120°.

2.1.1 The surgical method

The procedure is performed under general anesthesia. The patient is placed in the supine position on the operating room table, with the abdomen and groin sterilely prepped. The stomach is emptied with a suction catheter and the bladder using Crede maneuver, where older children are asked to urinate prior to entering the operating room. The ipsilateral hernia sac is reached through a skin-crease incision and simply dissected free from the adjacent tissue, the vessels and the spermatic cord and traced up to the internal ring. A reusable trocar is inserted through a longitudinal cut on the sac and secured in place with a suture (Figure 1).

The patient is then placed in the Trendelenburg position and the abdomen insufflated with CO_2, preferably at a low flow rate (1 l/min) to a maximum pressure of 8-10 mm Hg. The patency of the contralateral inguinal ring is assessed by the help of a 30-70°, 5 mm laparoscope. The positioning of the contralateral inguinal ring lies laterally to the lateral umbilical fold. The vas deferens in the male and the round ligament in female are traced over the pelvic brim to reach the internal inguinal ring. The presence of a significant peritoneal opening, the absence of an identifiable termination of the peritoneal sac, visualization of bubbles internally with external pressure, a hidden opening under a veil of peritoneum, a probing depth of 1.5 cm or concentric peritoneal rings distal to the internal ring are regarded as positive findings of patency (Figure 2).

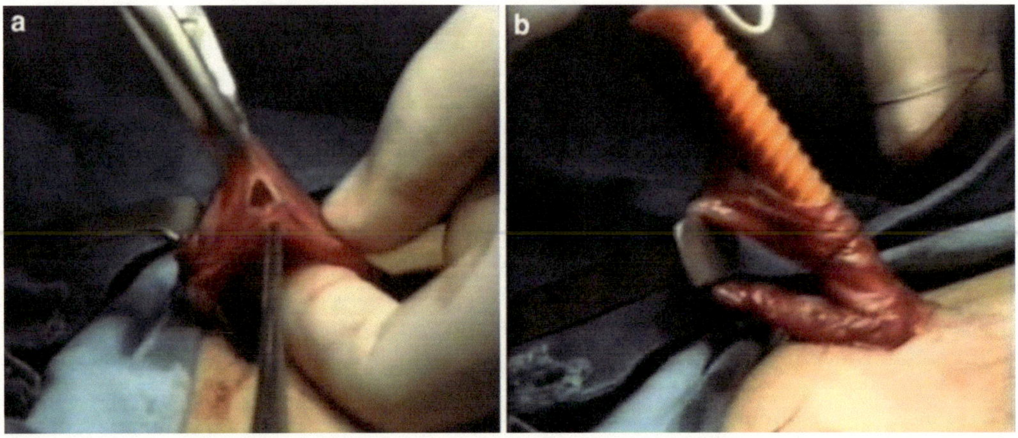

Fig. 1. Transinguinal approach to the contralateral side in unilateral hernia repair. Following insertion of a reusable trocar through the ipsilateral hernial sac, the port is secured in place with a suture.

A negative exploration means a flat or tenting peritoneal fold appearing as a shallow disk with a visible base at the internal inguinal ring (Figure 3). Herniotomy and high ligation is performed after decompressing the abdomen and terminating laparoscopy. In patients with a contralateral PPV, a simultaneous repair is accomplished.

The mentioned well-described surgical technique and the vast amount of scientific work established, however, have not yet defined the exact criteria in when to treat a patent processus vaginalis. It is a well-known fact that a standard description or method of assessment of a true PPV that may never present as a clinical hernia, is missing. Which is more confusing; Chan et al. had missed a rather shallow looking contralateral PPV in 1% of their cases during laparoscopic hernia repair, which later presented with a metachronous hernia[40]. Endo et al report a similar experience regarding six children in their series with a pinhole orifice or shallow depression, later presenting with metachronous hernia[36]. This fact poses quite an interesting contradiction to the generally adopted baseline probing depth of 1.5 cm. An interesting trend is that, higher PPV rates are increasingly reported recently, mostly due to the fact that laparoscopic repair is adopted in a wider number of institutions[40, 41, 52]. Endo et al. report that this difference is more than two fold. They state that such difference in PPV rates between the groups with diagnostic laparoscopy and laparoscopic hernia repair may be due to technical difficulties experienced during diagnostic laparoscopic examination[36]. Lau et al. report that 25–50% of the patients with a PPV, will present with a clinically significant hernia in the future[42]. Chung et al. support this perspective in their recent report, stating that the prevalence of asymptomatic PPV under laparoscopy is nearly twice the reported incidence of symptomatic contralateral hernia development after conventional unilateral herniotomy[43]. According to Maddox et al., 6.8% developed a metachronous hernia within a period of 53 months, amongst their study group presenting with 47.5% PPV[44]. This figure matches up closely with Miltenburg et al.'s meta-analysis[26].

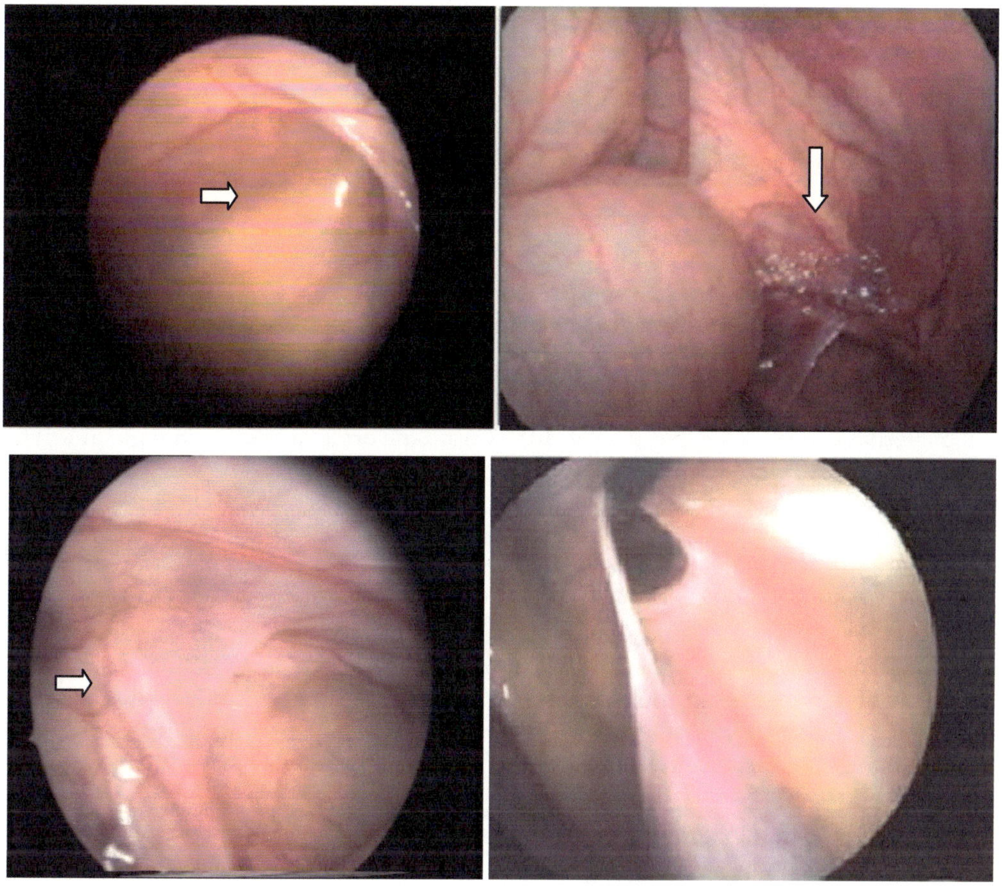

Fig. 2. Significant peritoneal opening on left side in female (upper left), visualization of bubbles on the left side in a male (upper right), obscure inguinal hernia under peritoneal veil on the right side (lower left), clearly visible peritoneal opening after drawing the veil away (lower right)

Apart from the discrepancy regarding the figures, diagnostic laparoscopy has certainly achieved its goal. It is obvious that we are sparing an increasing number of children less than 1 year of age, from routine exploration of their contralateral side. In other words, this simple examination prevents many unnecessary explorations. On the contrary, an increasing number of children over two years of age with a PPV were diagnosed and operated. Again, it is certain that these children will not present with a future hernia in the contralateral side.

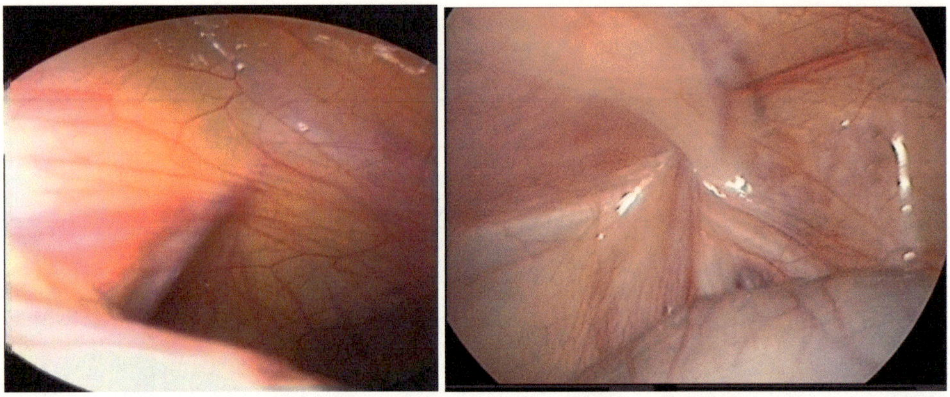

Fig. 3. Flat peritoneal fold on the right side in a male with no visible patency (left), tenting peritoneal fold on the left side in a male (right), both cases are regarded as PPV negative

3. Laparoscopic inguinal hernia repair in pediatric patients

The laparoscopic pediatric hernia repair is theoretically an identical alternate to the open technique. It is a reciprocal approach where the base of the hernia sac is ligated at the level of the internal inguinal ring, but mostly differs from the original open technique in leaving the sac in place. Albeit the described laparoscopic techniques, there is no single laparoscopic approach that has replaced the traditional repair[40-57]. The repair can be classified into two broad categories (intra or extraperitoneal) based on their approaches to the internal ring. The latter is mainly a subcutaneous endoscopically assisted ligation[40, 41, 53-55, 57]. All mentioned approaches require different types of suture material (absorbable nonabsorbable) as well as techniques of knotting (intracorporeal, extracorporeal) and wide range of endoscopic instruments (mainly required during extraperitoneal approach) are available[36, 41, 54, 58]. A highly disputable topic concerning feasibility of laparoscopic operations in an incarcerated inguinal hernia is beyond the limits of this chapter, and I do not recommended the reader unless having accomplished a good number of uncomplicated elective cases.

3.1 Laparoscopic inguinal hernia repair in female

The intraperitoneal approach requires increased skill in intracorporeal suturing and technical expertise to prevent jeopardy to the vas and testicular vessels. Thus, it may be justified to start practicing inguinal hernia repair in girls where there is limited risk of much feared collateral damage. In girls, a laparoscopic sac inversion and suture ligation or tying an endoloop at the base of the inverted sac, or excision and closure of the sac by placing a single purse string can all be practiced effectively[45, 56, 59-61]. Proponents of transcutaneous suturing methods advocate use of the technique in female as well[57, 58, 62].

3.1.1 The surgical method: Laparoscopic inguinal hernia repair in female using purse string

The procedure is performed under general anesthesia. The patient is placed in the supine position on the operating room table, with the abdomen and groin sterilely prepped. The stomach is emptied with a suction catheter and the bladder using Crede maneuver, where older children are asked to urinate prior to entering the operating room. An infraumbilical incision (open-Hasson technique) or a Veress needle is used in obtaining an abdominal access. Pneumoperitoneum is established with carbon dioxide according to appropriate age (8–10mmHg). Initially the abdomen is visualized using a 5-mm, 30° scope with the operating table positioned in moderate reverse Trendelenburg position. The pelvis is inspected for anatomical variations of the uterus, ovaries and adnex, and the inguinal rings are evaluated. Preferably two 2.7-mm working instruments are introduced through two lower abdominal stab incisions with (or without) the use of ports following detailed anatomic investigation. By the help of two grasping dissectors, the tip of the hernia sac is grasped and gently inverted into the abdominal cavity through the inguinal canal. One must be gentle with this blunt traction maneuver since brutal disruption of the distal attachments of the round ligament to the labia may lead to edema formation or extraperitoneal hemorrhage, which may render suturing of the neck of the inverted sac. When near or in the hernia sac, the fallopian tube and/or ovary are freed by a combination of blunt and sharp dissection. After confirming that the sac is relatively free of its surrounding attachments it is released back in place to continue with the purse string. The needle and thread are passed into the abdomen directly through the abdominal wall. By the help of a needle holder and grasping dissector, a 2-3/0 nonabsorbable monofilament purse suture is sewn just around the internal ring. In doing this, the suture must not cut deep in the surrounding tissue, to enable a strong and even strangling force on the peritoneal covering of the neck of the sac. The final bite is passed through the neck of the inverted sac. The suture is then secured at the base of the inverted hernia sac. It is advised to include sac resection after completion of suturing, since most published studies agree upon the fact that local peritoneal healing aids in preventing recurrences. A similar repair is applied to the contralateral side when indicated using the same incisions. Operation is terminated by removing all instruments under direct vision. The fascia and skin are closed with single Vicryl stitches. Stab incisions may be closed and dressed with Steristrips™ (3M; St. Paul, MN). A caudal block may additionally be used regarding parental consent. Otherwise, it is preferable to infiltrate all instrument or port sites prior to skin closure using local anesthetics. (All incisions are infiltrated with 0.25% or 0.5% bupivacaine solution) (Figures 4 & 5)

3.1.2 The surgical method: Laparoscopic inguinal hernia repair in female using endoloop

The procedure is almost identical to the method as previously described. High ligation of the inverted hernia may also be accomplished by the help of an Endoloop (Ethicon Inc., Somerville, NJ) which is completed by cinching down to the level of internal ring (Figure 6). According to published reports the average operating time overall is less than 40 minutes for bilateral repair, which is prolonged in premature infants and cases presenting with a sliding component such as incarcerated ovary. It is also reported that the simple use of endoloop may not be safe in patients presenting with large hernias and may require closure of the internal ring using laparoscopic intracorporeal suturing[56, 59]. Additional benefits of this procedure include diagnosis of androgen insensitivity and other dysgenic situations[45, 59, 60].

The protuberant mass of hernia sac 'rosebud' formed by the laparoscopic inversion and ligation method, is sonographically visible in all cases early after the procedure, has a characteristic appearance and gradually involutes with time[61].

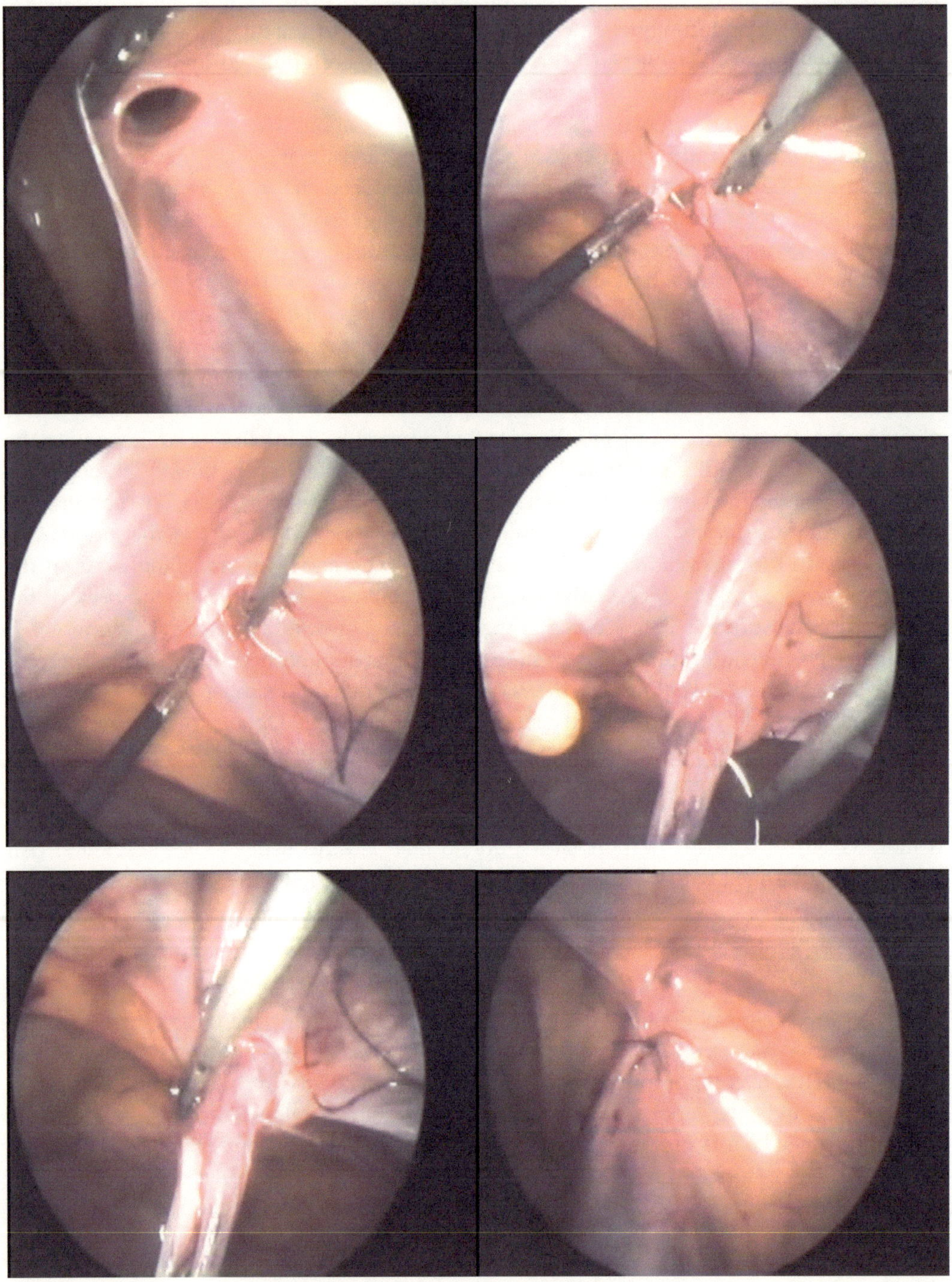

Fig. 4. Laparoscopic female hernia repair on the right side. Following placement of a purse suture around the internal ring, the final bite is passed through the neck of the inverted sac. The suture is than secured at the base.

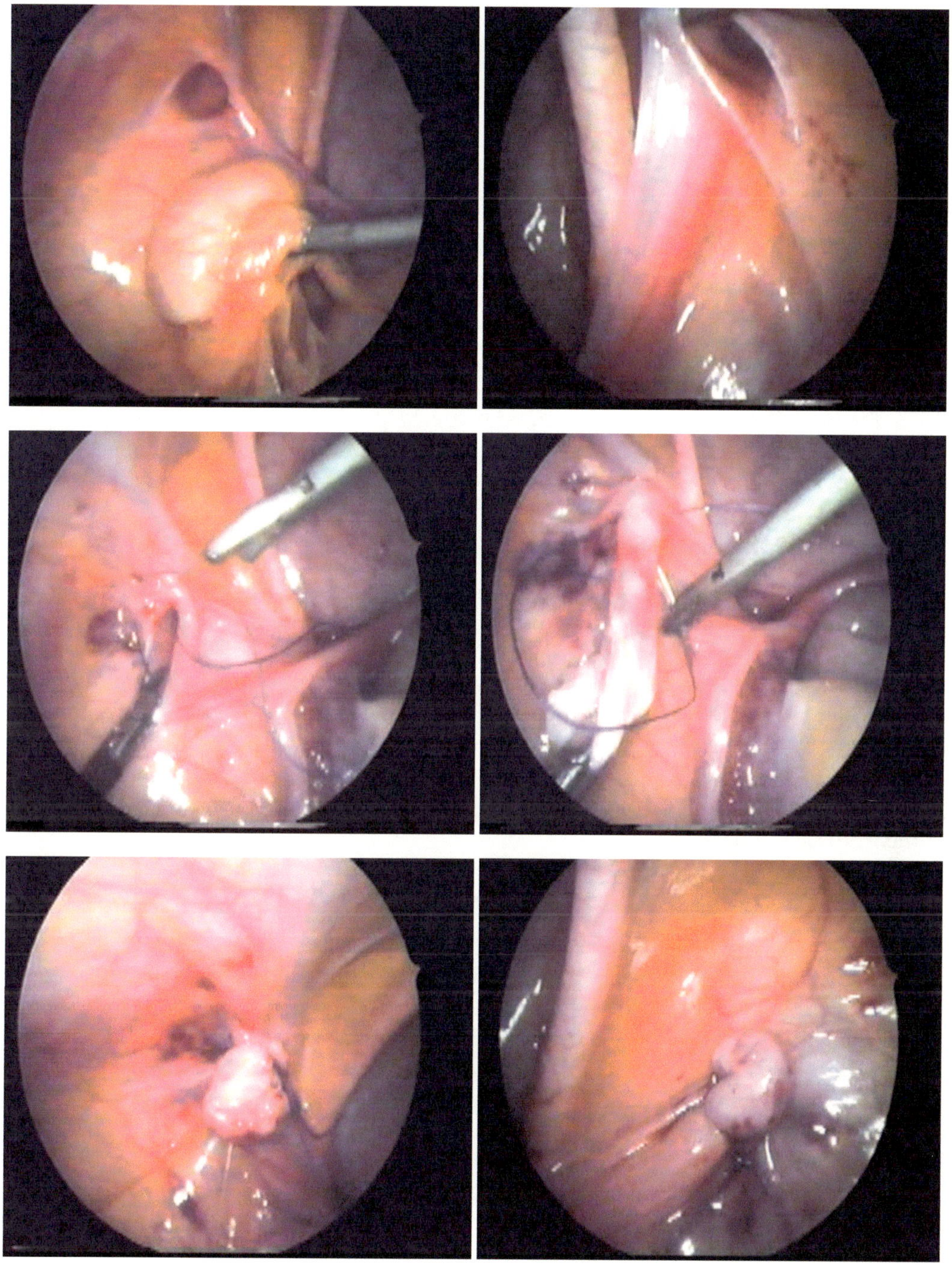

Fig. 5. Left inguinal hernia repair. Grasper is holding the left ovary (Top, left). During initial laparoscopic exploration, a PPV was found on the right side hidden under a peritoneal veil (Top, right). The operation was finalized as a bilateral repair. Looking at the result (bottom, right), we may speculate that this patient would have later come with a metachronous hernia, after a classic left hernia repair.

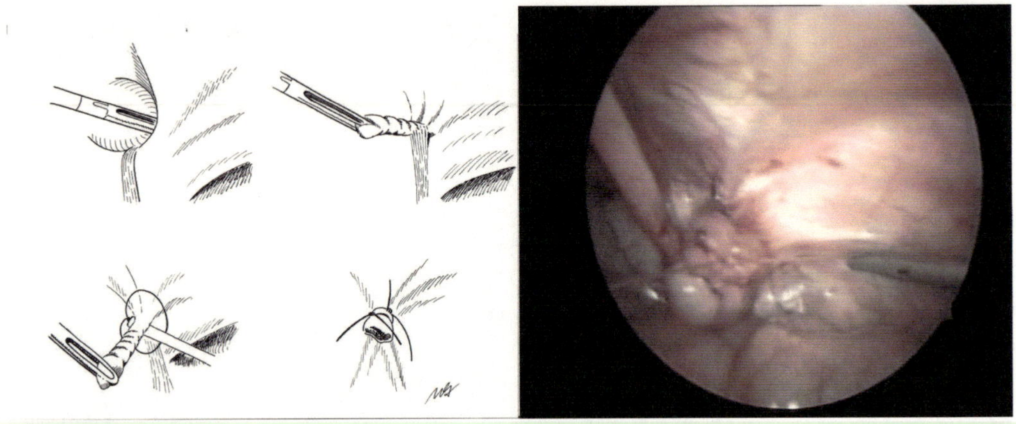

Fig. 6. The base of the inverted sac is secured by the help of Endoloop. Resection of the hernia sac is advised due to the fact that local peritoneal healing aids in preventing recurrences. "Rosebud" is seen on the right.

3.2 Laparoscopic inguinal hernia repair in male

The different techniques of laparoscopic repair have proven effective in males with equally good results. One may choose to close the peritoneal defect lateral to the cord using a purse string, Z-suture or interrupted sutures, either with or without the division of the continuity of the hernia sac. These techniques reproduce almost all the steps of open repair but without a groin incision. Unlike the technique used in female hernia repair, all variations of laparoscopic approaches in male are troubled with steep learning curves[42, 44-47, 50-52].

3.2.1 The surgical method: Laparoscopic inguinal hernia repair in male using intracorporeal suturing technique

The operation is performed under general anesthesia. The patient is placed in the supine position on the operating room table, with the abdomen and groin sterilely prepped. The stomach is emptied with a suction catheter and the bladder using Crede maneuver, where older children are asked to urinate prior to entering the operating room. Abdominal access may be gained either by an infraumbilical incision (open-Hasson technique) or by using a Veress needle. Pneumoperitoneum is established with carbon dioxide according to appropriate age (8–10mmHg). Initially the abdomen is visualized using a 5-mm, 30° scope with the operating table positioned in moderate reverse Trendelenburg position. The pelvis is inspected for anatomical variations such as Mullerian duct remnants and the inguinal rings are evaluated. Preferably two 2.7-mm working instruments are introduced through two lower abdominal stab incisions with (or without) the use of ports following detailed anatomic investigation. The needle and thread are passed into the abdomen directly through the abdominal wall. By the help of a needle holder and grasping dissector, a 2-3/0 nonabsorbable monofilament purse suture is sewn just around the internal ring. In doing this, the suture must not cut deep in the surrounding tissue, to enable a strong and even strangling force on the peritoneal covering of the neck of the sac. One must be careful to exclude all cord structures along the medial aspect of the internal ring. The needle is passed intraperitoneally just enough to bypass the vas/vessels, if it is not possible to dissect a plane between these structures. The suture is then secured at the base of the internal ring (Figures 7 & 8). Some authors advise to include semi circumferential sac incision on the antero-lateral aspect of the inguinal ring just distal to the purse string to aid in preventing recurrences. Operation is terminated by removing all instruments under direct vision. The fascia and skin are closed with single Vicryl stitches. Stab incisions may be closed and dressed with Steristrips™ (3M; St. Paul, MN). A caudal block may additionally be used regarding parental consent. Otherwise, it is preferable to infiltrate all instrument or port sites prior to skin closure using local anesthetics. (All incisions are infiltrated with 0.25% or 0.5% bupivacaine solution)

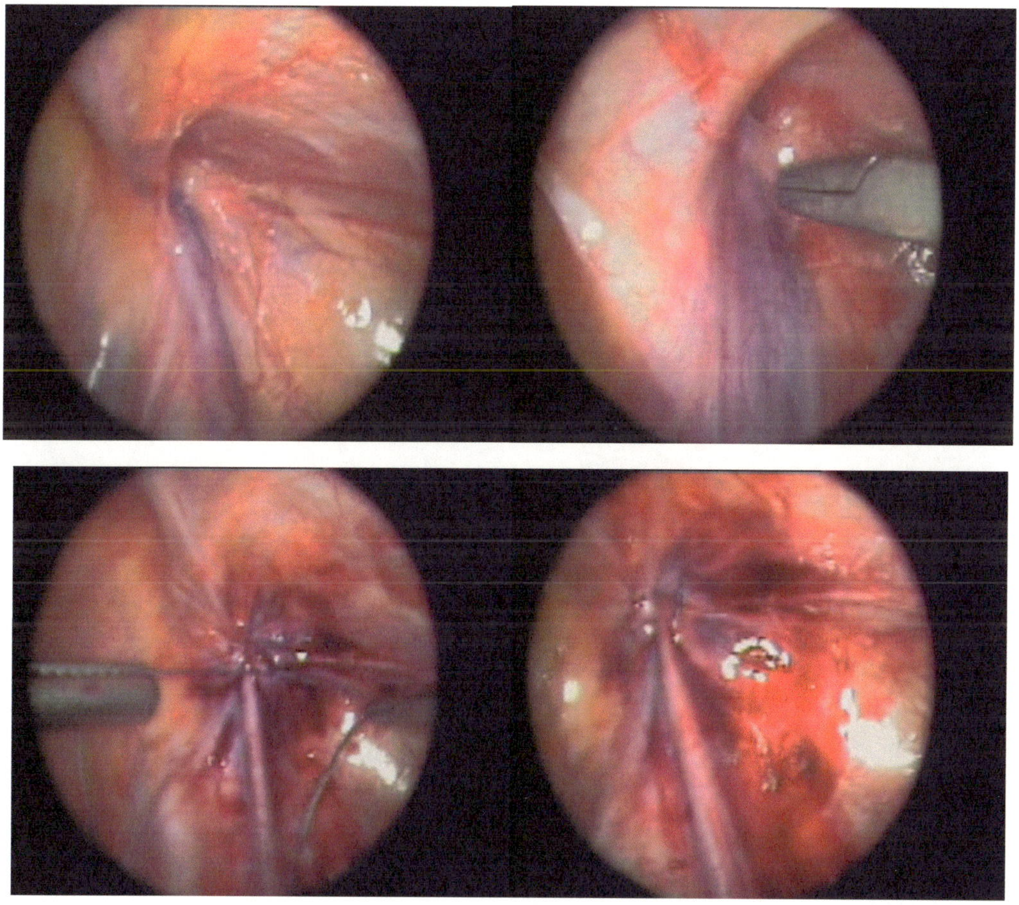

Fig. 7. Male hernia on the right. It is surprising to see such a small peritoneal opening in a patient who has presented with a big right inguinal hernia.

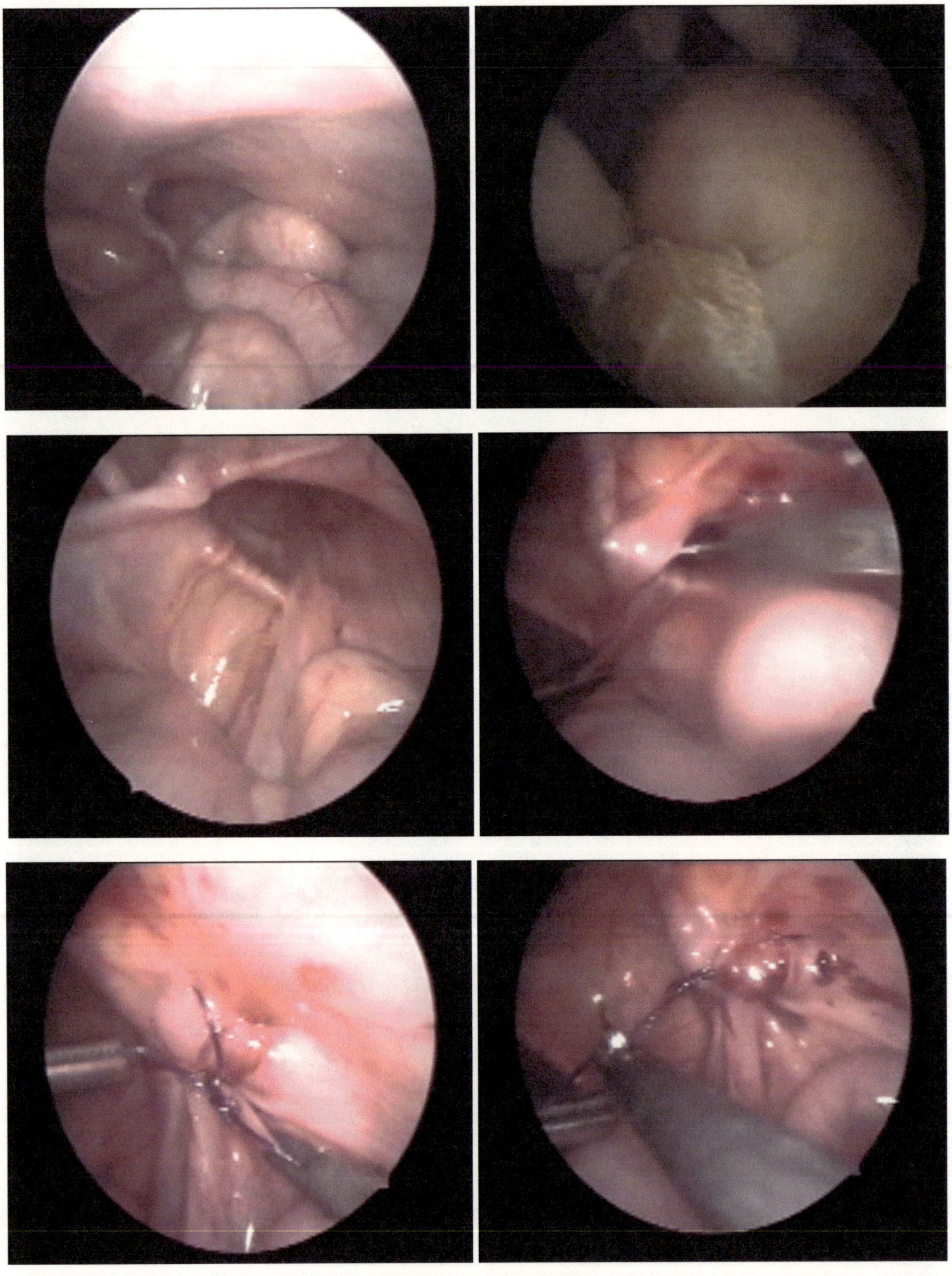

Fig. 8. A large scrotal hernia in male, with appendix in close proximity to the internal ring (Top left). The scrotum is filled with gas from an external view. (Top right). A purse string closes the defect effectively. In this case, stronger bites were taken from the margins.

The main point in repairing a male hernia obviously is to avoid damage to the vas and vessels. The needle or inclusion of these vital structures in the knot may cause injury; on the other hand, jumping over these structures to avoid them may lead to recurrence (Figure 9). An alternative technique involves raising a peritoneal flap by dissection and suturing it over the repaired defect. This is said to form a one-way peritoneal valve that prevents abdominal contents from entering the sac while selectively allowing fluid from the distal sac to enter the general peritoneal cavity, thereby preventing postoperative hydrocele formation[63].

3.2.2 The surgical method: Laparoscopic inguinal hernia repair in male using extracorporeal suturing technique

The patient is placed in a supine position and the entire abdomen and groin prepared into the field as described previously. The stomach is emptied with a suction catheter and the bladder using Crede maneuver, where older children are asked to urinate prior to entering the operating room. An infraumbilical incision (open-Hasson technique) or a Veress needle is used in obtaining an abdominal access. Pneumoperitoneum is established with carbon dioxide according to appropriate age (8–10mmHg). A 5-mm 30° laparoscope is introduced into the abdomen and both internal rings are inspected for hernial defects with the operating table positioned in moderate reverse Trendelenburg position. A 2-mm stab incision is made overlying the involved internal inguinal ring and the subcutaneous tissues are gently spread with a hemostat in order to bury the nonabsorbable knot. A nonabsorbable monofilament (preferably 2–0 Ethibond (Johnson & Johnson, Cincinnati, OH) suture on a CT-1 needle is then passed transcutaneously through this incision. The suture is passed just superficial to the peritoneum around the internal ring encircling the entire neck of the sac. Care must be taken to exclude all cord structures along the medial aspect of the internal ring. A 3-mm grasper instrument, inserted through a 2-mm stab incision in one of the lateral lower quadrants may be used only for manipulation of the vas deferens, spermatic vessels, and the peritoneal sac. In case of experiencing difficulty in dissecting a plane between the vas/vessels and the peritoneum, the needle must be passed intraperitoneally just enough to bypass the cord and vessel structures and then reintroduced into the extraperitoneal plane. The needle is then brought out partially through the skin; and once the swage of the needle is in the subcutaneous tissue, it is passed retrograde through the subcutaneous plane to be removed at the initial incision site. Do not forget to reduce pneumoperitoneum before tying up the knot. Authors recommend application of eight secure square knots while compressing the remaining insufflation gas from the hernia sac. The knot is buried beneath the original 2-mm stab incision, which may be approximated with an adhesive strip (Figure 10). A caudal block or local 0.25% bupivacaine may additionally be used as described previously.

The transcutaneous extracorporeal suturing technique is continuing to evolve. Chan and Tam advocate injection of extraperitoneal saline to lift the peritoneum off the underlying vas deferens and testicular vessels. They believe that the vas and vessels are protected by this maneuver, dissecting them free from the sac and leaving them in situ [49]. The proponents of this technique state that it only requires the use of extracorporeal knotting and decreases use of working ports and endoscopic instruments[36, 40, 41, 49, 53-55, 57, 62]. Initial reports of this technique showed a recurrence rate of 4.8%, infection, development of granuloma, and skin puckering at the site of a subcutaneously placed knot[36, 53, 58]. Recent reports however, declare the recurrence as 0.35%- 1.5%[40, 41, 62].

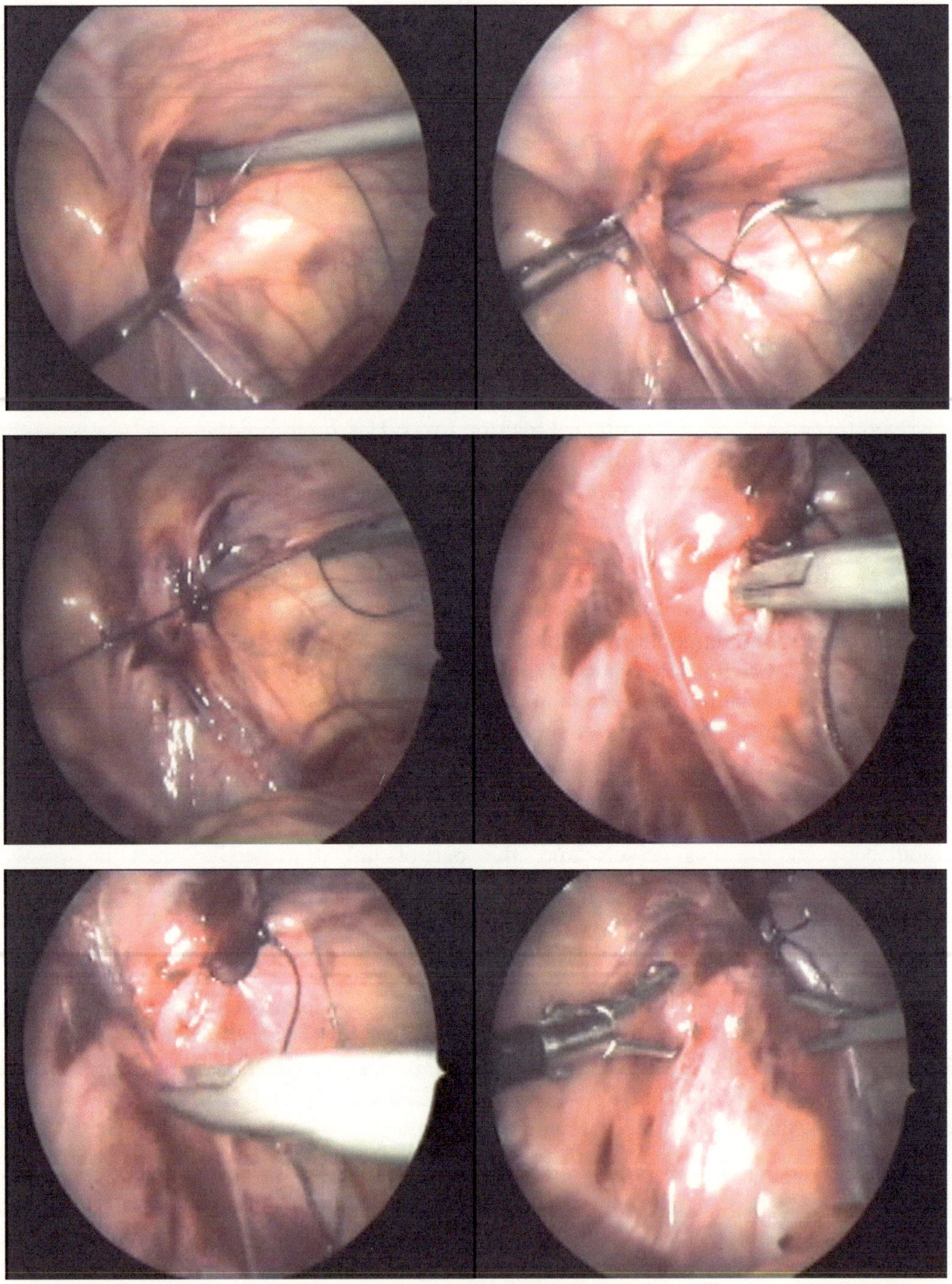

Fig. 9. Male inguinal hernia repair using Z suture technique. Small defect to the lateral needs additional suture (Middle left). Needle holder pointing the weak point where vas and vessels are (Middle right). Peritoneal fold to the left is used to cover the defect with additional suturing (Lower left).

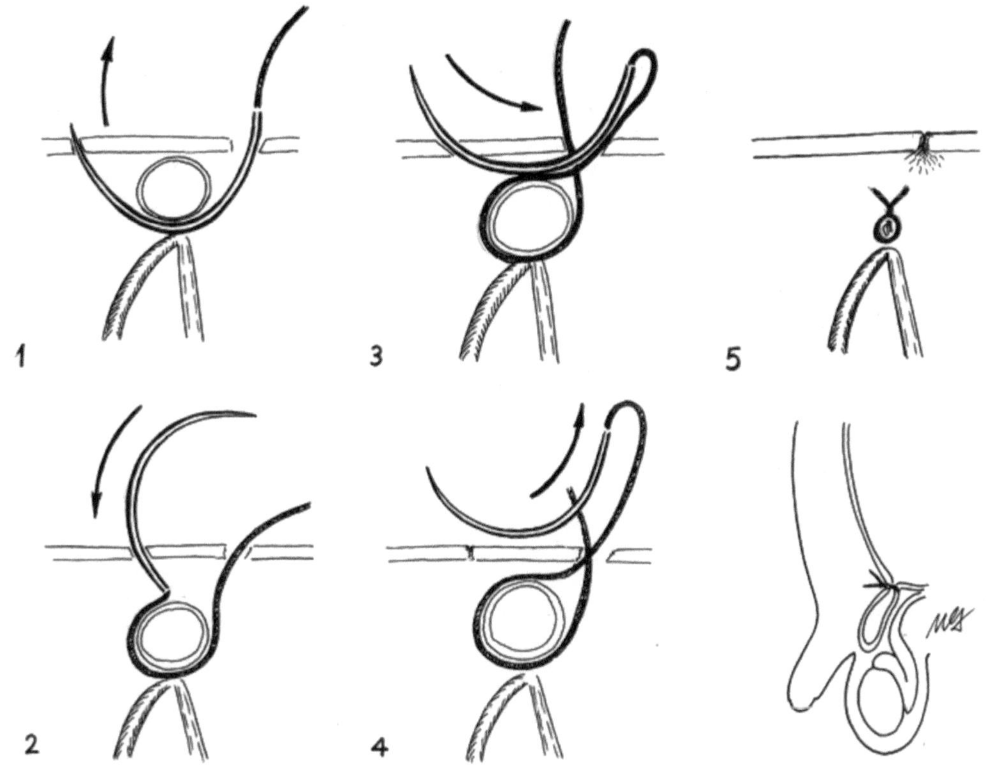

Fig. 10. The short operative time in extracorporeal suturing technique depends mostly on the knot tying method. It aids the surgeon feel comfortable and confident, using the same old familiar method in placing a suture. Those who would like to practice the method must remember that, crossing over the vas and vessels are not as easy as it seems in the figures.

4. Solving complications and contradictions

In contrast to the well-established laparoscopic inguinal hernia repair in the adult literature, a common laparoscopic hernia repair is still required to replace the traditional approach in pediatric inguinal hernia. This is mainly due to the steep learning curve in various introduced techniques and the reported troubling rates of recurrence.

The report on classic open repair with high ligation of the sac concerning 6361 patients by a single surgeon has excellent results with 1.2% recurrence rate, a 1.2% wound infection rate, and a 0.3% rate of testicular atrophy(64). Grosfeld has described the main factors affecting recurrence following common inguinal hernia repair, as failure to ligate the sac high enough at the internal ring, injury to the floor of the inguinal canal due to operative trauma, failure to close the internal ring in girls, and postoperative wound infection and hematoma(65). Classical repair entails higher recurrence risk for premature infants and incarcerated hernia, bearing high susceptibility to tearing during dissection of the thin and fragile hernia sac. Chan and Tam advocate laparoscopic technique as a method that can avoid all these possible causes of recurrence(49). In children omission of part of the ring circumference by jumping over vas/vessels, strength and appropriateness of the knot, inclusion of tissues other than peritoneum in the ligature with a propensity for subsequent loosening are reported factors that may contribute to recurrence. Additional factors are use of absorbable sutures, an excessively dilated internal ring, and the presence of comorbid conditions (eg, collagen disorders, malnutrition, or pulmonary disease). Most of the recurrences are noted within 6 months following the procedure and the most common site of recurrence is along the medial internal ring at the site of passage of the cord structures(51, 62, 66). The reported recurrence rates in extracorporeal suturing techniques are given between 0.35–2.8% in which small spaces are left when crossing over the spermatic cord or the testicular vessels(41, 54, 55, 57, 62). On the contrary, the reported recurrence rates 3.1–4.4% are much higher, in which the suture material is tied off in a similar way but intracorporeally(47, 52, 67). An intrinsic risk of recanalization of the vaginal process is mainly believed to result in recurrence. Albeit continuing search for a well-established approach in male repair, laparoscopic repair is becoming a promising good alternative to open hernia repair in female children. Comparable recurrence rates are repeatedly reported in female patients where the hernia sac is routinely excised(50, 59, 60).

The key to obtain a safe hernia repair relies on the healing process startled by firm ligation of the sac high enough at the internal ring, finally creating a good reperitonealization characterized by smooth and even surface like the palm of our hand. The optimum peritoneal tissue disruption is maintained by means of an essential bisecting force applied on the knot during tying it. This essential force must also warrant a good transfixation that would prevent the suture from migrating distally. A pediatric surgeon learns to feel and keep tactile control of this appropriate suture tension for obtaining an even bisecting and transfixating force. A time consuming, complex cognitive course is required to gain this tactile sense of feeling in hernia repair. The safety of a knot in a laparoscopic procedure relies on its limits in imitating an identical open procedure. What is meant by the "steep learning curve" is the surgeon's ability to regain expertise and persevere this mentioned, but new tactile feeling. The author believes that published better recurrence rates using extracorporeal suturing technique, depend on this familiar tactile sense of feeling and lower recurrence rates will equally be obtained with increased expertise in intracorporeal approaches. In the meantime, the use of double ligatures may further secure the closure of the hernia sac in intracorporeal approaches as well(41).

Published reports concerning impact of childhood hernia repair on fertility have always been a popular issue; it has forced proponents to restrict bilateral exploration according to the age and sex of the child and the presenting side(6-15). Antonoff et al. has pointed out to the higher risk of an inadvertent injury to vas deferens in the absence of a true hernia(68). Complications that may result in infertility during hernia repair include testicular atrophy, injury to the vas deferens, iatrogenic cryptorchidism, and injury to the fallopian tubes(3, 7, 15, 18, 40, 68-70). A recent survey declares a 5% infertility rate, medically diagnosed in males 50 years after hernia repair(71). Proponents of laparoscopic repair advocate the procedure arguing that the risk of visceral injury should be minimal or less than open surgery, keeping the vas deferens and cord un-touched by limited dissection of the peritoneal layer due to high visual magnifications(72). Theoretically, a laparoscopic approach aids the surgeon in avoiding a wide groin dissection thus reducing extensive inguinal scarring. The operative technique may also save the spermatic cord structures from a redo procedure related injury, should the hernia recur from a previous open repair(62). The reported rare incidence of testicular atrophy in laparoscopic hernia repair is attributed to multiple collateral circulations of the testis, rendering dissection at the internal ring an extremely safe method [73, 74]. Albeit reported advantages of pediatric laparoscopic hernia repair, the long-term risk of potential injury to the vas deferens and inguinal vessels should not be underestimated. Turial et al. reported 4% incidence of testicular ascent in babies weighing 5 kg or less, performed in skilled laparoscopic hands[75]. Yang et al. due to publishing bias, comment on the necessity of additional randomized controlled trials with standard report format and uniform units in order to investigate the efficiency of laparoscopic hernia repair with increased precision[76].

Other laparoscopy related complications such as; postoperative hydrocele, scrotal edema, erythema, inguinodynia and wound infections are reported decreasingly. Bharati et al. postulate that initial fluid accumulation in the distal sac recedes by spontaneous reabsorbtion and does not require any additional intervention[72]. In their recent meta-analysis report, Yang et al state that incidence of hydrocele, testicular atrophy, postoperative pain and wound infection show statistical insignificance, concerning laparoscopic vs. open hernia repair[76].

One must also admit that, laparoscopy carries its own set of complications such as decreased venous return, hypercapnia, acidosis and air embolism. Recent advancements in anesthesia and refinements in instruments have revolutionized use of minimal invasive approach as a safer procedure in pediatric surgical diseases[77]. On the other hand, intraperitoneal approach may additionally mean added risks associated with a violated peritoneal cavity inheriting specific complications caused by needle or trocar injury to ovary, bladder, intestines and/or the iliac, inferior epigastric and gonadal vessels. The burden of these risks is quite heavy to carry when compared to the common inguinal hernia repair. Laparoscopic approach, on the other hand, may also aid in finding an unexpected entity (Figure 11).

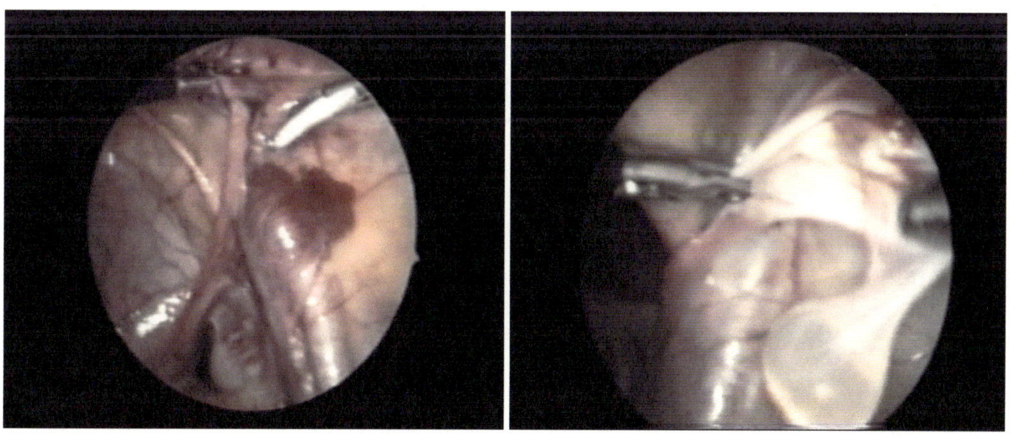

Fig. 11. An iatrogenic hematoma from a puncture in the internal iliac vein (Left). One must refrain from opening the retroperitoneum, since abdominal gas pressure is usually sufficient to stop the oozing. An intracanalicular cyst seen in a male patient, imitating the infamous Nuck's cyst in females (Right).

As for last but never the least, we have to evaluate the mentioned procedures by means of cost effectiveness. The long theater time required for the anesthetist in familiarizing with laparoscopic operations and for assembling all necessary equipment means a longer operative time, which in turn results in less operations in a day. When coupled with the high cost of setting up and running a theater with appropriate laparoscopic instrumentation, it may not be feasible, as it seems from an economic point of view.

5. Conclusion

It is certain that introduction of minimal invasive surgery has revolutionized the classical treatment of pediatric inguinal hernia repair, which has stood the test of time. Those who would think to commence are advised to do so from the initial step, diagnostic laparoscopy. Simple diagnostic laparoscopic examination enables surgical precision through enhanced visualization, magnification and ability to limit collateral damage by minimizing invasion. The reported incidence of a missed metachronous hernia following laparoscopic inspection is given as 1.1%, a figure far less than the expected traditional rate of a metachronous hernia(26, 36, 40). We may conclude that, a certain number of children will be saved from an unnecessary contralateral exploration or a future hernia by using this simple technique. We have to keep in mind; standards of management of a contralateral processus vaginalis awaits consensus.

Laparoscopic hernia repair is proven to allow easier access and excellent visual exposure to the detection and repair of contralateral patencies. The technique entails minimal manipulation of the vas deferens and testicular vessels during hernia repair, with suggested benefits of smaller scars, shorter bilateral operation times and better chance of repair of recurrent hernias through fresh tissue. Reported series however, still declare risk of higher recurrence and testicular ascent rates even in the most experienced hands. Again, it may be justified to start practicing inguinal hernia repair in girls where there is limited risk of much feared collateral damage. Albeit mentioned benefits, laparoscopic repair has potential risks attributable to surgeon's experience and variations in the chosen technique.

It is an important ethical duty for us to present the odds and evens and discuss the potential risks of each surgical approach with the family and have their consent during the decision making process.

6. Acknowledgment

The author would like to extend his gratitude to Mr. Mehmet Ali Gürsoy M.D. for drawing the illustrations within the text.

7. References

[1] Glick PL, Boulanger SC. Inguinal hernias and hydroceles. In: O'Neill JA, Rowe MI, Grosfeld JC, et al, editors. Pediatric surgery, 5th ed. St Louis, Mo: Mosby; 2007. p. 1172-92

[2] Weber TR, Tracy TF, Keller MS. Groin hernias and hydroceles. In: Ashcraft KW, Holcomb GW, Murphy JP, editors. Pediatric surgery. Philadelphia, Pa: Elsevier Saunders; 2005. p. 697-705

[3] Brandt ML. Pediatric Hernias. Surg Clin N Am 2008; 88: 27-43
[4] Kiesewetter WB, Parenzan L. When should hernia in the infant be treated bilaterally? JAMA 1959; 171: 287-90.
[5] Gilbert M, Clatworthy HW Jr. Bilateral operations for inguinal hernia and hydrocele in infancy and childhood. Am. J. Surg.1959; 97: 255-9.
[6] Shandling B, Janik JS. The vulnerability of the vas deferens. J Pediatr Surg 1981;16(4): 461-4.
[7] Janik JS, Shandling B. The vulnerability of the vas deferens (II): the case against routine bilateral inguinal exploration. J Pediatr Surg 1982;17(5):585-8.
[8] Abasiyanik A, Güvenç H, Yavuzer D, Peker O, Ince U. The effect of iatrogenic vas deferens injury on fertility in an experimental rat model. J Pediatr Surg 1997;32(8):1144-6.
[9] McGregor DB, Halverson K, McVay CB. The unilateral pediatric inguinal hernia: should the contralateral side be explored? J. Pediatr. Surg. 1980; 15: 313-7
[10] Given JP, Rubin SZ. Occurrence of contralateral hernia following unilateral repair in a pediatric hospital. J. Pediatr. Surg. 1989; 24: 963-5
[11] Tackett LD, Breuer CK, Luks FI, Caldamone AA, Breuer JG, DeLuca FG, Caesar RE, Efthemiou E, Wesselhoeft CW Jr. Incidence of contralateral inguinal hernia: a prospective analysis. J. Pediatr. Surg. 1999; 34: 684-7
[12] Ballantyne A, Jawaheer G, Munro FD. Contralateral groin exploration is not justified in infants with a unilateral inguinal hernia. Br. J. Surg. 2001; 85: 720-3
[13] Shabbir J, Moore A, O'Sullivan JB. Contralateral groin exploration is not justified in infants with a unilateral inguinal hernia. Ir. J. Med. Sci. 2003; 172: 18-9
[14] Ceylan H, Karakök M, Güldür E, Cengiz B, Bağci C, Mir E. Temporary stretch of the testicular pedicle may damage the vas deferens and the testis. J Pediatr Surg 2003;38(10):1530-3.
[15] Marulaiah M, Atkinson J, Kukkady A, Brown S, Samarakkody U. Is contralateral exploration necessary in preterm infants with unilateral inguinal hernia? J Pediatr Surg 2006;41(12):2004-7.
[16] Sparkman RS. Bilateral exploration in inguinal hernia in juvenile patients. Surgery 1962;51:393-406.
[17] Moss RL, Hatch EI. Inguinal hernia repair in early infancy. Am J Surg 1991;161:596-599
[18] Surana R, Puri P. Fate of patent processus vaginalis: A case against routine contralateral exploration for unilateral inguinal hernia in children. Pediatr Surg Int 1993;8:412-414
[19] Tackett LD, Breuer CK, Luks FI, Caldamone AA, Breuer JG, DeLuca FG, Caesar RE, Efthemiou E, Wesselhoeft CW Jr. Incidence of contralateral inguinal hernia: a prospective analysis. J. Pediatr. Surg. 1999; 34: 684-7
[20] Nakayama DK, Rowe MI. Inguinal hernia and the acute scrotum. Pediatr Rev 1989;11:87-93
[21] Rowe MI, Copelson LW, Clatworthy HW. The patent processus vaginalis and the inguinal hernia. J Pediatr Surg 1969;4:102-7
[22] Panton NM, Panton RJ. Laparoscopic hernia repair. Am J Surg 1994;167:535-537
[23] Watson DS, Sharp KW, Vasquez JM, Richards WO. Incidence of inguinal hernias during laparoscopy. South Med J 1994;87:23-25

[24] van Veen RN, van Wessem KJ, Halm JA, Simons MP, Plaisier PW, Jeekel J, Lange JF. Patent processus vaginalis in the adult as a risk factor for the occurrence of indirect inguinal hernia. Surg Endosc 2007;21(2):202–5
[25] Duckett J. W. Treatment of congenital inguinal hernia. Ann Surg. 1952 June; 135(6): 879–884
[26] Miltenburg DM, Nuchtern JG, Jaksic T, Kozinetz CA, Brandt ML. Meta-analysis of the risk of metachronous hernia in infants and children. Am J Surg 1997;174(6):741–4
[27] Erez I, Rathause V, Vacian I, Zohar E, Hoppenstein D, Werner M, Lazar L, Freud E.. Preoperative ultrasound and intraoperative findings of inguinal hernias in children: a prospective study of 642 children. J Pediatr Surg 2002;37(6):865–8
[28] Lobe TE, Schropp KP. Inguinal hernia in pediatrics: initial experience with laparoscopic inguinal exploration of the asymptomatic contralateral side. J. Laparoendosc. Surg. 1992; 2: 135–40
[29] Chu CC, Chou CY, Hsu TM, Yang TH, Ma CP, Cywes S. Intraoperative laparoscopy in unilateral hernia repair to detect a contralateral patent processus vaginalis. Pediatr Surg Int 1993;8:385-8
[30] Wolf SA, Hopkins JW. Laparoscopic incidence of contralateral patent processus vaginalis in boys with clinical unilateral hernias. J. Pediatr. Surg. 1994; 29: 1118–20
[31] Grossmann PA, Wolf SA, Hopkins JW, Paradise NF. The efficacy of laparoscopic examination of the internal inguinal ring in children. J. Pediatr. Surg. 1995; 30: 214–8
[32] Holcomb GW III, Morgan WM III, Brock JW III. Laparoscopic evaluation for contralateral patent processus vaginalis: part II. J. Pediatr. Surg. 1996; 31: 1170–3
[33] Yerkes EB, Brock JW 3rd, Holcomb GW 3rd, Morgan WM 3rd. Laparoscopic evaluation for a contralateral patent processus vaginalis: part III. Urology 1998; 51: 480–3
[34] Guvenc BH. Diagnostic laparoscopic evaluation of the contralateral internal inguinal ring: the search for a prospective hernia. Pediatr Endosurg Innov Techn 2001;5:259-65
[35] Miltenburg DM, Nuchtern JG, Jaksic T, Kozinetiz C, Brandt ML. Laparoscopic evaluation of the pediatric inguinal hernia: A meta-analysis. J Pediatr Surg 1998;33:874–879
[36] Endo M, Watanabe T, Nakano M, Yoshida F, Ukiyama E. Laparoscopic completely extraperitoneal repair of inguinal hernia in children: a single-institute experience with 1,257 repairs compared with cut-down herniorrhaphy. Surg Endosc. 2009 Aug;23(8):1706-12.
[37] Sözübir S, Ekingen G, Senel U, Kahraman H, Güvenç BH. A continuous debate on contralateral processus vaginalis: evaluation technique and approach to patency. Hernia 2006; 10: 74–8.
[38] Fuenfer MM, Pitts RM, Georgeson KE. Laparoscopic exploration of the contralateral groin in children: An improved technique. J Laparoendosc Surg 1996 (suppl 1):S1–S4.
[39] Owings EP, Georgeson KE. A new technique for laparoscopic exploration to find contralateral patent processus vaginalis. Surg Endosc 2000;14:114–116.
[40] Chan KL, Chan YH, Tam PKH. Towards a near-zero recurrence rate in laparoscopic inguinal hernia repair for pediatric patients of all ages. J Pediatr Surg 2007;42:1993-7.
[41] Tam YH, Lee KH, Sihoe JD, Chan KW, Wong PY, Cheung ST, Mou JW. Laparoscopic hernia repair in children by the hook method: a single-center series of 433 consecutive patients Journal of Pediatric Surgery 2009; 44, 1502–1505.

[42] Lau ST, Lee YH, Caty MG. Current management of hernias and hydroceles. Semin. Pediatr. Surg. 2007; 16: 50-7.
[43] Maddox MM, Smith DP. A long-term prospective analysis of pediatric unilateral inguinal hernias: should laparoscopy or anything else influence the management of the contralateral side? J. Pediatr. Urol. 2008; 4: 141-5
[44] Chung KLY, Leung MWY, Chao NSY, Wong BPY, Kwok WK, Liu K KW. Laparoscopic repair on asymptomatic contralateral patent processus vaginalis in children with unilateral inguinal hernia: A centre experience and review of the literature Surgical Practice 2011; 15: 12-15
[45] Montupet P, Esposito C. Laparoscopic treatment of congenital inguinal hernia in children. J Pediatr Surg 1999;34(3):420-3.
[46] Tan HL. Laparoscopic repair of inguinal hernias in children. J. Pediatr. Surg. 2001; 36: 833
[47] Schier F, Montupet P, Esposito C Laparoscopic inguinal herniorrhaphy in children. A three-center experience with 933 repairs. J Pediatr Surg 2002; 37:395-397
[48] Yip KF, Tam PK, Li MK. Laparoscopic flip-flap hernioplasty: an innovative technique for pediatric hernia surgery. Surg Endosc 2004;18(7):1126-9
[49] Chan KL, Tam PK. Technical refinements in laparoscopic repair of childhood inguinal hernia. Surg Endosc 2004; 18:957-960
[50] Becmeur F, Philippe P, Lemandat-Schultz A, Moog R, Grandadam S, Lieber A, Toledano D. A continuous series of 96 laparoscopic inguinal hernia repairs in children by a new technique. Surg Endosc 2004; 18:1738-1741
[51] Chinnaswamy P, Malladi V, Jani KV, Parthasarthi R, Shetty RA, Kavalakat AJ, Prakash A. Laparoscopic inguinal hernia repair in children. JSLS 2005; 9:393-398
[52] Schier F. Laparoscopic inguinal hernia repair: a prospective personal series of 542 children. J Pediatr Surg 2006; 41:1081-1084
[53] Ozgediz D, Roayaie K, Lee H, Nobuhara KK, Farmer DL, Bratton B, Harrison MR. Subcutaneous endoscopically assisted ligation (SEAL) of the internal ring for repair of inguinal hernias in children: report of a new technique and early results. Surg Endosc 2007;21(8):1327-31
[54] Spurbeck WW, Prasad R, Lobe TE. Two-year experience with minimally invasive herniorrhaphy in children. Surg Endosc 2005; 19:551-553
[55] Patkowski D, Czernik J, Chrzan R, Jaworski W, Apoznanski W. Percutaneous internal ring suturing: a simple minimally invasive technique for inguinal hernia repair in children. J Laparoendosc Adv Surg Tech 2006; 16:513-517
[56] El-Gohary MA. Laparoscopic ligation of inguinal of inguinal hernia in girls. Pediatr Endosurg Innov Techn 1997;1:185-7
[57] Takehara H, Yakabe S, Kameoka K. Laparoscopic percutaneous extraperitoneal closure for inguinal hernia in children: clinical outcome of 972 repairs done in 3 pediatric surgical institutions. J Pediatr Surg 2006; 41:1999-2003
[58] Prasad R, Lovvorn HN 3rd, Wadie GM, Lobe TE. Early experience with minimally invasive inguinal herniorrhaphy in children. J Pediatr Surg 2003;38:1055-8
[59] Lipskar AM, Soffer SZ, Glick RD, Rosen NG, Levitt MA, Hong AR. Laparoscopic inguinal hernia inversion and ligation in female children: a review of 173 consecutive cases at a single institution. Journal of Pediatric Surgery (2010) 45, 1370-1374

[60] Guner YS, Emami CN, Chokshi NK, Wang K, Shin CE. Inversion herniotomy: a laparoscopic technique for female inguinal hernia repair. J Laparoendosc Adv Surg Tech A. 2010 Jun;20(5):481-4

[61] Akansel G, Guvenc BH, Ekingen G, Sozubir S, Tuzlaci A, Inan N. Ultrasonographic findings after laparoscopic repair of paediatric female inguinal hernias: the 'vanishing rosebud'. Pediatr Radiol. 2003 Oct;33(10):693-6

[62] Dutta S, Albanese C. Transcutaneous laparoscopic hernia repair in children: a prospective review of 275 hernia repairs with minimum 2-year follow-up. Surg Endosc 2009; 23:103–107

[63] Yip KF, Tam PK, Li MK. Laparoscopic flip-flap hernioplasty: an innovative technique for pediatric hernia surgery. Surg Endosc 2004;18(7):1126–9

[64] Ein SH, Njere I, Ein A. Six thousand three hundred sixty-one pediatric inguinal hernias: a 35-year review. J Pediatr Surg 2006;41(5):980–6

[65] Grosfeld JL, Minnick K, Shedd F, West KW, Rescoria FJ, Vane DW. Inguinal hernia in children: factors affecting recurrence in 62 cases. 1991; J Pediatr Surg 26:283–287

[66] Kastenberg Z, Bruzoni M, Dutta S. A modification of the laparoscopic transcutaneous inguinal hernia repair to achieve transfixation ligature of the hernia sac Journal of Pediatric Surgery 2011; 46, 1658

[67] Chinnaswamy P, Malladi V, Jani KV, Parthasarthi R, Shetty RA, Kavalakat AJ, Prakash A. Laparoscopic inguinal hernia repair in children. JSLS 2005; 9:393–398

[68] Antonoff MB, Kreykes NS, Saltzman DA, Acton RD. American Academy of Pediatrics section on surgery hernia survey revisited. J Pediatr Surg 2005;40(6):1009–14

[69] Hansen KA, Eyster KM. Infertility: an unusual complication of inguinal herniorrhaphy. Fertil Steril 2006;86(1):217

[70] Matsuda T, Muguruma K, Hiura Y, Okuno H, Shichiri Y, Yoshida O. Seminal tract obstruction caused by childhood inguinal herniorrhaphy: results of microsurgical reanastomosis. J Urol 1998;159(3):837–40

[71] Zendejas B, Zarroug AE, Erben YM, Holley CT, Farley DR. Impact of childhood inguinal hernia repair in adulthood: 50 years of follow-up. J Am Coll Surg. 2010 Dec;211(6):762-8

[72] Bharathi RS, Arora M, Baskaran V. Minimal access surgery of pediatric inguinal hernias: a review. Surg Endosc 2008;22:1751-62

[73] Barqawi A, Furness III P, Koyle M. Laparoscopic Palomo varicocelectomy in the adolescent is safe after previous ipsilateral inguinal surgery. BJU Int 2002;89:269-72

[74] Riccabona M, Oswald J, Koen M, Lusuardi L, Radmayr C, Bartsch G. Optimizing the operative treatment of boys with varicocele: sequential comparison of 4 techniques. J Urol 2003;169:666-8

[75] Turial S, Enders J, Krause K, Schier F. Laparoscopic inguinal herniorrhaphy in babies weighing 5 kg or less. Surg Endosc. 2011 Jan;25(1):72-8

[76] Yang C, Zhang H, Pu J, Mei H, Zheng L, Tong Q. Laparoscopic vs open herniorrhaphy in the management of pediatric inguinal hernia: a systemic review and meta-analysis. Journal of Pediatric Surgery 2011; 46, 1824–1834

[77] Ozdamar D, Güvenç BH, Toker K, Solak M, Ekingen G. Comparison of the effect of LMA and ETT on ventilation and intragastric pressure in pediatric laparoscopic procedures. Minerva Anestesiol. 2010; Aug;76(8):592-9